THE LITERARY LIFELINE

THE LITERARY LIFELINE

Bibliotherapy and the Transforming Power of Reading

KEVIN HARVEY

BLOOMSBURY ACADEMIC
LONDON • NEW YORK • OXFORD • NEW DELHI • SYDNEY

BLOOMSBURY ACADEMIC
Bloomsbury Publishing Plc, 50 Bedford Square, London, WC1B 3DP, UK
Bloomsbury Publishing Inc, 1385 Broadway, New York, NY 10018, USA
Bloomsbury Publishing Ireland, 29 Earlsfort Terrace, Dublin 2, D02 AY28, Ireland

BLOOMSBURY, BLOOMSBURY ACADEMIC and the Diana logo are trademarks of Bloomsbury
Publishing Plc

First published in Great Britain 2025

Cover design: Ben Anslow
Cover image © Trinity Mirror / Mirrorpix / Alamy Stock Photo

A catalogue record for this book is available from the British Library.

Library of Congress Cataloging-in-Publication Data
Names: Harvey, Kevin (Sociolinguist), author.
Title: The literary lifeline : bibliotherapy and the transforming power of reading / Kevin Harvey.
Description: London, UK ; New York, NY, USA : Bloomsbury Academic, 2025. |
Includes bibliographical references and index. | Summary: "The Literary Lifeline is a tribute to the
transporting and consoling power of reading. Interweaving fragments from his own experience of
reading, Harvey takes us on a fascinating tour of reading for therapeutic effect, exploring the rise of
shared reading and other uses of bibliotherapy in various social and personal contexts. He argues,
through a series of compelling stories and life experiences, that reading not only benefits physical
and emotional wellbeing, but that it also humanises the care process, particularly in institutional
settings where personhood can be threatened or undermined completely"– Provided by publisher.
Identifiers: LCCN 2024051064 (print) | LCCN 2024051065 (ebook) |
ISBN 9781472583598 (HB) | ISBN 9781472583604 (PB) |
ISBN 9781472583611 (ePDF) | ISBN 9781472583628 (eBook)
Subjects: LCSH: Bibliotherapy.
Classification: LCC RC489.B48 H37 2025 (print) | LCC RC489.B48 (ebook) |
DDC 615.8/5162–dc23/eng/20250407
LC record available at https://lccn.loc.gov/2024051064
LC ebook record available at https://lccn.loc.gov/2024051065

ISBN: HB: 978-1-4725-8359-8
PB: 978-1-4725-8360-4
ePDF: 978-1-4725-8361-1
eBook: 978-1-4725-8362-8

Typeset by Newgen KnowledgeWorks Pvt. Ltd., Chennai, India

For product safety related questions contact
productsafety@bloomsbury.com.

To find out more about our authors and books visit www.bloomsbury.com
and sign up for our newsletters.

In loving memory of Clive (brother much missed)

CONTENTS

ACKNOWLEDGEMENTS

Many people have helped me during the preparation of this book. First and foremost, thanks to my editors (past and present) at Bloomsbury: Gurdeep Mattu, Andrew Wardell, Morwenna Scott, Elizabeth Holmes, Jasmine Paul, Laura Gallon and Sarah MacDonald. I'm especially grateful to Laura and Sarah, who, when the finish line grew closer, heroically tolerated my endless entreaties, and without whom I would never have delivered the manuscript on time, if at all. I would also like to thank Balasuwathiga and team at Newgen for their assiduous production work.

For their encouragement, insights and permissions, thanks to: David Bevan, David Day, Jenny Denton, Jenny Day, Chris Ward, Elaine Harvey, Julie Harvey, Malcolm Harvey, Gareth Breen, Rosa Sanchez Panchuelo, David Jolly, Anne Oxborough, Raymond Tallis, Ben Masters, Blake Morrison, Andrew Motion, Philip Davis, Jane Davis, Julie Walker, Liz Brewster, Ella Berthoud, Alan Bennett, Sue Sanderson, Gavin Francis, Sam Jordison, Paul Stanbridge, John Fuller, Lucy Jones, Christina Lee, Daniel Hunt, Malgorzata Chalupnik, Gavin Brookes, Graham Caveney, Rebecca Peck, Graeme Docherty, Andrew Harrison, Chris Collins, Louise Mullany, Mike Jones, Thorlac Turville-Petre, Joe Jackson, Jim Moran, Nicola Royan, Tom Dening, Surinder Bangar, Svenja Adolphs, Máire ní Fhlathúin.

Thanks also to Susan Jones, Dave Peplow, Dave Beddow, Jenny Hills (and fellow shared reading facilitators and group members), all of whom have shaped my thinking about what it means to be a reader.

Lastly, and most importantly, I want to thank Ana for her kindness and understanding, and Mae for her unwavering enthusiasm. ('What's your book about, Daddy?' 'Reading.' 'Who wants to read a book about reading?')

Copyright Acknowledgements

Every effort has been made to trace copyright holders and to obtain their permission for the use of copyright material. However, if any have been inadvertently overlooked, the publishers will be pleased, if notified of any omissions, to make the necessary arrangement at the first opportunity.

Excerpt from Alan Bennett's 'Diary: What I Did in 2015' in the *London Review of Books* by permission of the author.

Excerpt from Alison Moore's *He Wants* by permission of Salt Publishing.

D. H. Lawrence's 'Self-Pity' from *The Cambridge Edition of the Works of DH Lawrence: Poems* by permission of the estate of Frieda Lawrence Ravagli and Cambridge University Press.

Excerpt from Dorothy P. Holinger's *The Anatomy of Grief* by permission of Yale University Press.

Extracts from Edward Parnell's *Ghostland* by permission of HarperCollins.

Excerpt from Gillian Clarke's 'Miracle on St David's Day' from *Collected Poems* by permission of Carcanet Press.

John Killick's 'Freedom' from *Creativity and Communication in Persons with Dementia* by permission of Jessica Kingsley Publishers.

Extracts from John Masefield's *The Box of Delights* by permission of HarperCollins.

Laurie Sheck's 'Mysteriously Standing' from *Captivity* by permission of Penguin Random House.

Extract from 'Last Song' by Miguel Hernández (author) and A. S. Kline (translator), copyright 2007.

Excerpt from Paul Standbridge's *My Mind to Me a Kingdom Is* by permission of the author and Galley Beggar Press.

Extracts from Roland Barthes's *Mourning Diary* by permission of Notting Hill Editions.

Stanza from Roy Fuller's *Ghost Voice* by permission of London Magazine Editions.

Excerpt from Robert D Richardson's *Three Roads Back: How Emerson, Thoreau, and William James Responded to the Greatest Losses of Their Lives* by Princeton University Press.

Robert Frost's 'The Road Not Taken' from *The Poetry of Robert Frost* edited by Edward Connery Lathem. Copyright © 1928, 1969 by Henry Holt and Company. Copyright © 1956 by Robert Frost. Reprinted by permission of Henry Holt and Company. All Rights Reserved.

Excerpt from W. S. Graham's 'Dear Bryan Wynter' by permission of Faber & Faber.

PREFACE

This is a partial and lopsided book. (Off to a good start then.) My intention had been to write a monograph that rigorously and compendiously explored the relationship between literature and health. But as I began to research and write the book, I realized that not only was this an impossible undertaking (impossible for me at least), but that other books had since been published on the topic – the kind of books (rigorous, compendious) that I could never hope to write.

Despite these setbacks, there were still things I wanted to say about the restorative power of reading. And besides, I had a contract to fulfil. Consequently, the book changed shape and direction. It became more wide-ranging, more tangential and more personal – less a monograph in the end than a collection of free-standing pieces touching on themes as varied as the state of public libraries, poetry and dementia, notebook reflections on personal loss and grief, doctors who write, senior living complexes, shared reading and reading aloud, and the language of health and illness. These resultant pieces don't 'hang grandly together', to borrow a phrase from Galen Strawson, but they do connect in potentially meaningful ways.

Each of these pieces is broadly concerned with the transformative potential of reading. It is hardly original, of course, to claim that reading changes lives. But I have long been fascinated by the social and therapeutic use of literature, the contribution that poetry, plays and fiction can make to improving health and quality of life, particularly in the context of reading aloud and shared reading. Recent times have witnessed a proliferation of participatory reading activities: it is estimated, for example, that over 600 shared reading groups now operate across the UK, taking place in settings as varied as schools, hospitals,

homeless shelters, libraries, drug rehabilitation centres and prisons. The rise
and impact of these community reading programmes has been described – not
unjustly – as a 'reading revolution', 'bringing great writing to life and putting
good reading into the hands of people who need it'.

In the opening piece, 'The reading revolution: Shared reading and reading
for well-being', I examine the rise of shared reading groups and the growth
of participatory reading. Described by Blake Morrison as 'one of the most
heartening phenomena of our time', shared reading brings people together
from all walks of life to read aloud and enjoy literary texts – a format that is
fundamentally different from the traditional reading group in which people
meet to talk about books read in advance. The emphasis in shared reading is on
the experience of texts being read aloud in real time, and on the ensuing open
and open-minded discussions that emerge from the live reading experience.
('For once a week we're all on the same page', said one of the participants in
a prison reading group I observed. 'We're no longer prisoners. We're people
again.')

Apart from the social facets of shared reading, I also consider the effects
that the activity has on emotional and physical well-being. The therapeutic
benefits of shared reading derive not only from the experience of people
coming together but also from the immersive reading of literature. Paying
close attention to and discussing literary texts has been shown to help people
with chronic pain separate themselves from their physical discomfort,
and to help people with depression recover their emotional equilibrium.
Literature, in the inimitable words of Philip Davis, acts as a 'trigger' or
'rocket-boost' – 'reaching levels of emotion, memory, and recognition not
normally available or easily accessible in daily life'. The kind of immersive
thinking that takes place in shared reading groups 'goes deeper than
therapeutic step-by-step programmes' – intriguingly, the very fact that
shared reading is not top-down therapy, Davis argues, makes it all the more
'freely therapeutic'.

If shared reading is avowedly non-top-down therapy, other modes of reading for well-being are more standardly therapeutic in their delivery and approach. In the final part of the piece, I consider the rise of bibliotherapy, including schemes such as the popular books on prescription service, along with other forms of prescribed reading. Although there is a large body of research demonstrating the health and social benefits of shared reading, less is empirically known about much of the various forms of bibliotherapy available to the public. I consider the evidence around bibliotherapy interventions for health and well-being, opening up questions about its mechanics, what people get out of it, and why they turn to it in the first place.

The second piece, 'What have libraries ever done for us? In defence of the public library system', is a personal and autobiographical essay reflecting on the current state of the public library. It seems absurd to have to mount a defence of free education and book provision, along with all the information and social resources that libraries make available. But since 2010, because of austerity measures implemented by the then Tory-led British government, almost one-fifth (almost 800) of the UK's public libraries have shut down – a pace of decline that evokes, in John Sutherland's chillingly memorable phrase, 'extinction rather than evolution'. The closures come at a time when there is a huge disparity in adult literacy across the UK, with, according to the National Literacy Trust, one in six adults in England having very poor literacy skills. The continued dismantling of the public library also comes at a time when the UK is recovering from the social and economic fallout of the Covid pandemic, which has only widened the attainment gap between the advantaged and the disadvantaged.

As a child I had little interest in reading, and even less in libraries (fusty, boring old places). It was only later in life, and almost entirely by accident, that I began to appreciate the blessings of the public library. I was a disaffected 23-year-old police constable who happened to stumble upon Nottingham's Angel Row Library. The library was the perfect place for a restless copper to hang out, a gateway to worlds far more exciting and enriching than my own. An inexperienced reader, I picked at the shelves at first, but soon set about them with increasing urgency and momentum, to the point of obsessive abandon, believing that somewhere among all those books and pages was the secret to 'my full, true story'. The library became an emotional and intellectual refuge, a virtual second home. I would sometimes spend almost entire shifts there, devouring book after book, at the expense of pursuing petty thieves and shoplifters as I was supposed to be doing.

Some fifteen years later, long after I'd made good my escape from the police, I paid a return visit to Angel Row. The trip was more than just a nostalgic amble down memory lane: I wanted to know how the place was faring in times of austerity, to assess the impact of funding cuts on its services. It was also an opportunity to observe the library's day-to-day running and activities (so much of what happens in libraries – the children's reading schemes, the adult literacy groups, the language cafes, the job seekers' support sessions, the mental health reading groups, and all those innumerable private, personal epiphanies – is immune to the crude measurement of footfall, the quantitative metric commonly used to gauge the value of public library systems). Spending time speaking to staff and patrons, watching the daily goings-on at Angel Row, only convinced me that libraries are just as much about social capital as they are about silence and reflection, places where it is possible to reconcile the need for social contact with the need for solitude and seclusion. Government closures will certainly save money in the short term but, as I argue, will cost communities dearly in the end.

The next two pieces return to the theme of reading for well-being, but specifically in the context of dementia care. Much has been written about the therapeutic effect of music, how, with its ability to reach subcortical regions of the brain, it enhances cognition in people with dementia. But what about reading – the reading of poetry in particular? Poetry, as with music, exploits recurring accents and patterns, sounds structured in and through time. In the first of these two pieces, 'Poetry and the new culture of dementia care', I consider some of the ways in which poetry produces restorative and quickening effects in readers, writers and listeners, how it triggers recollections and recovers moods, fostering social and emotional well-being.

As with music and other arts therapies, poetry therapy is a relatively recent approach to dementia care. Arts-based approaches are part of what has been described as a new culture of care, a culture that no longer regards people with dementia as leftover 'husks' or 'shells' of their former selves but recognizes their potential for growth and development. In keeping with the tenets of the new culture, I argue that it is still possible for people with dementia, even advanced dementia, to maintain a sense of self and personal identity.

This is a theme I develop in the following piece, 'The enduring self: A journal', an account of my time spent reading poetry aloud to Robert, a retired lecturer of English literature living with Alzheimer's disease. Although Robert's cognitive function was severely affected by the disease, the reading took him out of himself, away from the confines of his sheltered accommodation, back to the seminar room and lecture theatre. He was the expert again, attuned to the music and meaning of the poems, assured and responsive. The more time I spent with Robert, the more I came to question the assumption, widely held in Western philosophical thought, that self-consciousness is the yardstick of personal identity, that 'the continuity of self-consciousness … makes us the persons we are'. There was little doubt that Robert failed to meet this strict hyper-cognitive criterion – and yet, all the same, his responses to the poems, his laughter, his gestures and all his other embodied behaviours expressed a purposive sense of being in the world, a subtly realized selfhood.

The penultimate piece, 'The doctor as writer, the writer as doctor', finds me in conversation with general practitioner and acclaimed author Dr Gavin Francis. Along with Henry Marsh, Rachel Clarke, Atul Gawande, Joanna Cannon and others, Francis is one of a new generation of doctor-authors exploring the intersection between literature and medical science (Francis is also a very astute reader). For these doctors, medicine is storytelling: storytelling as an act of witness, a way of being open to and honouring the lives of their patients. They are all compelling authors – writers with a canny facility for stringing together the dual narratives of doctor and patient, for plumbing the space between sickness and health.

When I spoke with Francis in December 2019, shortly before the publication of his fifth book *Island Dreams*, I wanted to know more about his approach to storytelling. I wanted to know how being an author affected his relationship with his patients, and how he balanced his twin roles of writer and general practitioner. Did he think of himself more as an author than a doctor, and did he believe that being a writer made him a better practitioner, better able to read his patients? The interview was also an opportunity to talk to Francis about his development as an author and his acquaintance with the great John Berger, whose book *A Fortunate Man*, a masterpiece of medical biography, though long out of print, Francis had been instrumental in helping to republish.

The final and longest piece takes the form of a notebook-diary I kept following the death of my brother in April 2022. He was forty-eight, my brother, my first friend and my best friend, and I loved and miss him very much. Keeping a notebook, no matter how short and fragmented the entries were, was a way of trying to make sense of his death, an attempt to put into words what seemed so beyond the reach of words. ('You learn,' writes Chimamanda Ngozi Adichie, 'how much grief is about language, the failure of language and the grasping for language.')

Keeping a notebook was also a means of reflecting on the language of illness, particularly metaphor and other figurative devices. So much of the talk about my brother's cancer was freighted with metaphors depicting it in moral and military terms – a battle he could win if he was prepared to fight hard enough (whatever 'fighting' and 'fighting hard enough' precisely entailed). For much of the time, particularly in the immediate wake of his diagnosis, I didn't know what to say to him. How often did I skirt his questions about the futility of it all and resort to specious arguments and mollifying conceits? I once told him – as though I knew all about these things and had the right to tell him – that to be close to death was to be truly authentic, consecrated, and therefore, paradoxically, to be more vitally alive. (Quite the consolation.)

Increasingly, when I was able to, I found myself turning to literature – in particular, the poetry of Thomas Hardy and Denise Riley, writers unswervingly fluent in the language of loss. I learned from them not so much how to grieve or how to handle loss but – and this was something by no means obvious to me at the time – how grief has 'to be done', 'to be expressed' and the pain endured. I found the poems unbearable at times, impossible for all kinds of reasons. But over time they, and insights from other writers, helped to bring a tentative kind of peace. Not a calming or reassuring peace but a peace born of the assurance that what we have known and experienced 'cannot disappear as if it had never been'.

December 2024

1

The reading revolution:
Shared reading and reading
for well-being

The ideal reader must learn how to listen.
– ALBERTO MANGUEL

Come and take choice of all my library and so beguile thy sorrow.
– WILLIAM SHAKESPEARE

The reading revolution

I keep forgetting I'm in jail.

It's only when I catch sight of the small, steel-barred window high up in the wall that I remember where I am. But no sooner do I register the bars than I slip back into the wider world of the novel we're reading. Those bars apart, this could be any shared reading group.

We're approaching the end of the story, a climax as terrible as it is compelling. I know what's coming. So, evidently, do the men.

'Emotion's took over him – he's not thinking clearly.'

'You can imagine his face.'

'Lots of darkness in the description, isn't there?'

'The dark rim of the woods.'

'The colour highlights his desperation.'

'That impending sense of doom – the loss to come.'

'I just feel so sorry for the lad.'

But there's humour too.

'Those brambles are terrible!' one of them remarks. 'I think everyone's had a bramble moment.'

As the laughter subsides and the reading resumes, I think of the hundreds of other men here in the prison, wonder what they're doing at this moment, how they're filling time, the interminable hours …

In prison, time is the enemy. Prison time, writes Claude Lucas, 'doesn't move toward any horizon; it gapes. A gaping abyss that must be filled at any cost.' Unlike the countless hours spent alone in their cells – dead time, gaping time – the time spent here together in the reading group, the men tell me, is sacred, time meaningfully spent. It's 'an oasis', one of them says, adding that there's no way he would have finished the novel had he been reading it alone in his cell.

The men take it in turns to read. They read for about five to ten minutes each. Not all of them read, but most do, and do so confidently. Some read with considerable relish and panache, pausing to maintain suspense and generate surprise; others intone dialogue in a variety of different voices, often to the amusement of fellow group members. (All of which reminds me that every act of reading aloud is a performance, a far from passive interpretation of the words on the page.)

Towards the end of the session, the group moves on to poetry. As Lyndsay, the group facilitator (from The Reader Organisation at the University of Liverpool), hands out a selection of poems, the men let out a mild groan, begrudging the switch in genre. ('Poetry's boring,' one of them mutters.) But when Lyndsay begins to recite the poems, their faces unfrown, and a tolerable attention supervenes. At any rate, they all seem to follow the reading; some even nod and smile at the text, silently mouthing certain words over and over to themselves, as if encountering them for the first time. And on the occasions when Lyndsay pauses to elicit responses from the group (as is customary in shared reading) the men fall to discussing the form of the poems, eager to tease out meanings and probe authorial intentions, posing the kind of questions that wouldn't be out of place in one of my university seminars.

But what strikes me most is how intimate the talk is. In between their more literary-critical exchanges, the men share personal stories and emotions, reflecting on their time in prison and their former lives outside. The reading evidently provides a safe confessional space for the men, who continually refract their experiences through the reading, translating it into the terms of their own predicaments. ('If you went to a group of ten prisoners,' Lyndsay tells me later, 'and asked them to tell you about their lives, they'd clam up. But if you read a book together – the text is a kind of proxy, a medium through which they can talk about themselves.') When the session finishes, I notice how most of the men, despite their professed dislike for poetry, fold up their handouts and discreetly tuck them into their trouser pockets.

Outside the group, the men, I learn, like to read thrillers and true crime – not the kind of staple that features in the weekly shared reading sessions. The Reader is strict about its choice of reading matter. Its shared reading model is premised on what it calls 'great' and 'serious' literature – a veiled reference to the canon, to the tradition of English letters. Accordingly, it's out with James Patterson and Marian Keyes, and in with Shakespeare and Carol Ann Duffy. Or to put it another way: it's no to popular and genre fiction – detective stories, 'chick lit' and so on – and yes to literary fiction and poetry.

Yet it would be wrong to suggest that The Reader shuns popular texts. 'It's not true that we only read serious or great literature', says Jane Davis, the organization's founder and director, whom I met not long after my visit to the prison. 'We have to respond to the situation where people are. If you said to me, "You're going to work with this nineteen-year-old single mum with three kids", I'd be mad to take A*nna Karenina* along on the first meeting.' For Davis, establishing tastes and interests, getting to know people, is more important than plunging straight into the text. And if doing so involves reading Kim Kardashian's biography, so be it. Making the connection comes first. Once you've made that connection, she says, then you can think about unleashing Tolstoy.

Davis's passion for introducing people to shared reading, for bringing people and books together, goes back to her days in adult education over twenty-five years ago, when she was teaching extramural classes at the University of Liverpool. In her candid autobiographical essay, 'Something Real to Carry Home When the Day Is Done', she describes how, during the later part of her twenty years as a literature teacher, she began to feel that something was missing from her life, that she needed 'something else'. She wasn't sure what that something was, only that it would have something to do with literature, which, for her, had been 'both a life-saver and life-giver'. When she was growing up, reading was more than a pastime, more than a source of entertainment and information. In the face of parental neglect ('Mum was usually in the pub and my father was not around'), books were life: not only did they afford mental escape, they offered meaning and connection – clues about how to live. 'I read literature as myself, through my own eyes, trying to apply it to my own life and my own moral problems.'

After becoming a university teacher and settling into a life that would have been unimaginable without the input of literature, Davis increasingly began to feel that 'this life-giving resource was not being harnessed by people who might have great need of it':

Things crystallised one day when I was driving to university to teach Wordsworth's 'Ode: Intimations of immortality'. It was spring and there were daffodils lining the path to the door of an ex-council house opposite the traffic lights where I had stopped in North Birkenhead. The daffodils were dancing, and the door was opened by a younger woman in her pyjamas with a baby, perhaps a year old on her arm. He seemed to leap up with joy at the sight of the older woman, and I thought, 'the babe leaps up on her mother's arms', a line from the Immortality Ode I had been reading earlier that day. At exactly the same moment that the line came into my mind, a thought also exploded: that child will never read Wordsworth. He'll never think 'the babe leaps up' or know 'The Daffodils'. He can't have this stuff that has made a life for me. He will get a bad education, not including any of the joy and usefulness of poetry, and he'll end in a dead-end job, or in prison, and be hurt by life. The light changed and I drove off. Within months, I'd set up a five-week summer outreach project called 'Get Into Reading'. The first session took place in a community centre on the other side of that set of lights.

**

Who knows whether any of the prisoners I met had read Wordsworth? None of them, at any rate, professed a great love for poetry. And yet one of the main reasons why they attended the reading group was to encounter new texts and ideas, to be introduced to books they hadn't read before, to genres to which they weren't typically accustomed. They spoke of their desire to be challenged, to be drawn out of their comfort zones, to embrace fresh perspectives. They spoke about the distracting influence of television ('when TVs came along, I stopped reading'), but how, each week, shared reading brought them back to books ('which do things to you that TV doesn't'). They spoke about the alliance among them, how being part of the reading group encouraged them to open up and share different, conflicting points of view. Reading and responding to texts together brought them closer, made them stronger: 'It's the bond that counts. For once a week we're all on the same page. We're not in prison. We're no longer prisoners. We're people again. Reading leads to other things.'

In many ways, the prison reading group perfectly encapsulates the work of The Reader. Whatever the setting – criminal justice, drugs and alcohol rehabilitation, mental health, residential care – the chief virtue of shared reading is its inclusiveness, its ability to engage with hard-to-reach and socially excluded groups. Shared reading makes reading a 'creative, social, life-enhancing activity', provides opportunities for participants to build skills and confidence, to extend their prospects and horizons. Various surveys have shown that shared reading improves well-being, and that people feel better for reading together. Some have even described the activity as a lifeline, crediting it with easing them back into society and reawakening their interest in life.

Although The Reader has grown exponentially since its beginnings and has done a tremendous amount of good, Jane Davis, who is nothing if not ambitious, wants shared reading to go further, to enter into the mainstream. She wants to see shared reading take place in public libraries across all parts of the UK. She wants to see it integrated more fully into public health, for it to become a staple feature of social prescribing for psychological well-being, as readily available as more traditional treatments such as medication and talking therapies.

Prescribed shared reading, she concedes, might not be to everyone's taste. But it offers an alternative response to emotional healing. She speaks here of people who regularly seek help from their GP – those experiencing social and economic exclusion or emotional and existential crises – but for whom conventional medicine has little to offer, people whose lives have become, as she puts it, 'stuck'.

'Doctors,' she explains, 'can't fix a lot of human stuck-ness. Which isn't to say that it isn't the right thing for people to have anti-depressants or CBT, etc. Of course it is. Of course. But it's not enough – it's not a varied enough offer, because often what people need is human connection, a reason to get up in the morning, and something interesting to have their mind on.'

Giving it out loud

For the last ten years or so, I've helped to run a community reading group (inspired by, and conceived along the lines of, The Reader's shared reading model). We're a small, intimate group that meets once a week in the lobby of a local church. The lobby is the nerve centre of the place, a hub of civic activity – all lunch clubs and friendship groups – and the ambient noise often makes it difficult to read aloud. But it's good to be part of the busy collective: it amplifies the liveness of the moment, the sense of shared experience.

The group is made up of a set of regular members but is open to anyone. People often join us after stopping by the church for a hot meal and shelter. Rather than return directly to the streets, they linger a while, tentatively take a handout before pulling up a chair and sitting with us around the table. Some return in the following weeks; others we never see again. At the time of writing, the group consists of eight regular members, who range from kitchen porters and supermarket staff to retired teachers and servicemen. Each has their reason for attending: some crave the company, others value the contemplative space the weekly meetings afford – though all share a love of the spoken word, and delight in encountering unfamiliar texts, no matter how obscure or difficult (though we've yet to tackle the poetry of J. H. Prynne).

Much of the joy of reading aloud comes from the act of sharing – 'the mingling of emotions as the work unfolds', as Oliver Edwards puts it. Initially, however, I think some of the group members found the experience of shared reading aloud a little awkward, partly because the activity was alien to them but mainly because of my difficulty animating the words on the page.

Back then, I was an unpractised reader aloud. Other than reading bedtime stories to my two-year-old daughter, I'd had little experience of reading aloud to others. I was perfectly able to do *Where the Wild Things Are* in different grunts and bellows, but when I read aloud to the group, no matter how I tried to vary my voice, I struggled to recover the timbre and rhythmic sense of the words. For all intents I was reading silently, reading, that is, with the eyes and not for the ear. Rather than give each word its due, I would slide over and chunk words together, taking the kind of syntactic leaps and short cuts one is prone to make when processing language internally. It wasn't simply that I read too quickly (though going more slowly would've helped). It was more that I was conflating my inner voice with my outer voice, and in doing so failing to convey the essential flavour of the text.

My struggle to hone an effective reading voice only served to illustrate how accustomed we have become to silent reading, how we have lost the art of reading aloud. In his book *Beyond Good and Evil*, Friedrich Nietzsche reminds us that reading aloud used to be the norm (up until the tenth century at least), lamenting the rise and eventual ascendancy of silent reading. The modern reader, he opines, 'has put his ears away in the drawer. In antiquity, when a man read – which he did very seldom – he read to himself aloud, and indeed in a loud voice; it was a matter for surprise if someone read quietly, and people secretly asked themselves why he did so.' The 'loud voice' to which Nietzsche here refers is not so much a stentorian voice, as a voice with

all the crescendos, inflections, variations of tone and changes of tempo in which the ancient public world took pleasure. In those days the rules of written style were the same as those of spoken style; and these rules depended in part on the astonishing development, the refined requirements of ear and larynx, in part on the strength, endurance and power of ancient lungs.

For Nietzsche, the lungs of antiquity were far superior to their modern counterparts: 'We have really no right to the grand period, we moderns, we who are short of breath in every sense!' Whether ancient lungs, physiologically speaking, were better conditioned to reading aloud is a moot point. But Nietzsche's account of reading in classical times highlights something we tend to overlook about reading aloud, namely, the physical and emotional demands it places on the reader. It can be exhausting! When, to take an extreme example, Charles Dickens gave his famous public readings of his works, his heart rate shot up dramatically. During a reading aloud from *Oliver Twist* at St James's Hall on 15 February 1870, his pulse increased from 72 to 124, a leap of 52 beats a minute. The reading so depleted Dickens that afterwards he had to be assisted to his dressing room, where he collapsed on a sofa, unable to speak 'a rational or consecutive sentence' for a full ten minutes.

(Dickens put everything into his readings. As he scowled and grimaced, shrieked and bellowed, he became his characters, vicariously experiencing their violence and aggression, their terror and distress. 'I shall tear myself to pieces', he whispered to his friend Charles Kent as he went on-stage to give his heart-racing performance of *Oliver Twist*. Four months later, Dickens collapsed again and died the following day without regaining consciousness. (Official cause of death: 'apoplexy'.))

Apoplexy notwithstanding, I tried for a while to emulate Dickens's delivery. It was a way of gingering up my performance, a way of attempting to resolve the ongoing conflict between my inner voice and outer voice. Like Dickens, I did all the different characters. But try as I might, I was too self-conscious to do them with any real staginess or conviction – to give myself over completely to the performance. To read aloud is to expose oneself to the scrutiny and judgement of others, to risk trying your audience's patience, and sometimes when I was reading to the group, I would suddenly think, My God, I'm reading aloud – I'm reading aloud to people! – and my voice would falter and the blood come up, and the words would start to feel heavy, each one a burden, more weight than word – it was as if the text was pressing down on me and I was having to hold it up, to push it away – and it was all I could do to sound the words, to distinguish one word from another, let alone voice them with any kind of sentential inflection or variation of tone. Only by relinquishing the text, reciting it without thought or understanding, was I able to keep on going;

otherwise, my voice would freeze completely, bringing me to a mortifying standstill.

Even now, many years later, I still experience problems getting the words out: an unexpected parenthesis or embedded clause might wrong-foot me, or a looming expletive, winking in the distance, pitch me into a state of quavering anticipation. But nowadays I'm less anxious about getting it wrong. Over the years I've become a more confident reader, better able at least to weather my mistakes, and have grown to enjoy the performatory aspect of reading aloud, the challenge and pleasure of raising others 'to the level of the book'.

What I feel more than anything when I read aloud now is not so much anxiety (though it's still present in some mild form) as gratitude and appreciation. 'In reading aloud, you are greatly privileged,' writes Holbrook Jackson, 'first to consort with all that is noble and beautiful in thought and imagination, and then to give it forth again.' I love the intimate dialogue with the author that reading aloud affords, how it forces you to see deeply 'into the words and patterns of words'. Unlike silent reading, where 'only the writer performs', reading aloud is always a collaborative, interpretive process. You create and occupy a world together. You become, as Jackson puts it, a spokesperson and intermediary for the author, add your voice to their voice, your vision to theirs, your two minds becoming one.

Special thinking

When I first got involved in shared reading, I was a university tutor of some seven years' standing. Throughout my academic career, I'd become accustomed to reading and analysing texts from an impersonal, critical standpoint. I was used to treating texts as ideological constructs, networks of discursive representations and practices – things, at any rate, that needed to be pulled apart to expose the assumptions behind them. In lectures and seminars,

I inducted eager undergraduates into the ways of textual critique, taught them how to flush out a discourse and pull binary oppositions apart. I laid down strict interpretative parameters. It wouldn't really do to second-guess the author or frame one's responses in intuitive, evaluative terms, to stray too far from the text. If my students 'transgressed' in this way, I would gently reign them in, return them to the path of critical righteousness, for I knew better.

But shared reading has little in common with the kind of reading and discussion that takes place in a critical studies seminar. My shared reading participants – these so-called 'ordinary readers' – were untrained in the art of deconstruction. They brought a happy anarchy to the page, to the raw experience of reading, against which my critical theories and beloved metalanguage afforded little hermeneutic protection. I had no formula for dealing with people's instinctive, emotional responses, which were often deeply personal and sometimes blissfully unpredictable.

Not long after the group first got together, we read Seamus Heaney's 'Blackberry Picking'. In this poignant early poem, Heaney describes, in rich sensuous detail, the childhood delights of foraging for blackberries, along with the attendant realization that the youthful adventure, beauty and hope of the experience will inevitably end with the rotting of the fruit. The final line of the poem – which I read aloud slowly, solemnly, drawing out the caesura between the words 'keep' and 'knew' for dramatic emphasis – is as follows:

Each year I hoped they'd keep, knew they would not.

There followed a long contemplative silence before Rita, not usually the first to initiate conversation, and without the slightest hint of irony, observed:

Well, he should've put them in the freezer.

Rita's response, I thought rather scornfully, was hardly likely to redefine and expand the boundaries of Heaney studies. If I'd encountered such a remark in one of my academic seminars, I'd have sidestepped it completely, deemed it immaterial to the exegetical task at hand. And yet there was something terrifically liberating about Rita's response. As an 'untrained' reader she had, to borrow John Bayley's phrase, no 'standardised technique' for dealing with the poem and hence no need to supply her own 'ready-made lock-up' for herself and the text to occupy. She was untroubled by what appeared on the page, unencumbered by any notion of relevance or correctness. In the context of shared reading, her remarks served to illustrate the various ways in which different meanings, judgements and personal associations are brought to the discussion of literary texts. Shared anecdotes based on the storage of soft fruit across different families, times and regions ensued from Rita's comments – anecdotes which in turn led to further personal stories and disclosures, both related and completely unrelated to the poem. (But oh, how I longed to drag them back to the materiality of the text, to some phrase or image ripe for critical picking!)

This propensity for storytelling and self-disclosure became one of the hallmarks of the group. Over time, their accounts and anecdotes, triggered by the texts we were sharing, became more and more personal, more and more private. A reading of Tony Harrison's poem 'Timer', an affecting reflection on the death of the poet's mother, prompted one group member, a man in his eighties who seldom discussed his personal life, to speak at length about the passing of his own mother and his dazed participation in the events that followed her death ('why wasn't she there to help me?'). During a discussion of Carol Ann Duffy's 'The World's Wife', another regular group member, who often regaled us with her unfailingly sunny tales of domestic and family life, was moved to share her experience of living with an abusive partner and her 'constant struggle to keep up appearances'. On such occasions, as with the prison reading group, it felt as though the participants were just as much speaking through the texts as for themselves, their lifeworlds and emotions intimately tied to the words on the page.

***

What was it exactly that brought about this confessional – and evidently cathartic – effect? Doubtless the live communal reading and social dynamics of the group played a part. But what was it about the texts themselves – the literature – that opened up thought and feeling? The literary scholar Josie Billington, who has written extensively on shared reading and well-being, argues that the expressive potential of literature, its language of release, affords the 'right emotional atmosphere in which to hear and speak' and 'to explore inner life'. Literature generates for the reader a felt situation, enabling 'thoughts to be thought that might not otherwise find a place for themselves; thoughts that, like their thinkers, might not ever quite fit in to any contemporary framework'. This kind of thinking is by no means smooth and easy, or straightforwardly consoling; it is often intense and demanding, involving as it does a struggle to articulate ideas and truths that one might otherwise wish to suppress.

Billington provides many prime examples of readers thinking through literature. One of the most illuminating involves a group reading of Robert Frost's American classic 'The Road Not Taken', a poem concerned, among other things, with the problem of moral choice.

Two roads diverged in a yellow wood,
And sorry I could not travel both
And be one traveler, long I stood
And looked down one as far as I could
To where it bent in the undergrowth;

Then took the other, as just as fair,
And having perhaps the better claim,
Because it was grassy and wanted wear;
Though as for that the passing there
Had worn them really about the same,

> And both that morning equally lay
> In leaves no step had trodden black.
> Oh, I kept the first for another day!
> Yet knowing how way leads on to way,
> I doubted if I should ever come back.
>
> I shall be telling this with a sigh
> Somewhere ages and ages hence:
> Two roads diverged in a wood, and I –
> I took the one less traveled by,
> And that has made all the difference.

One of the group participants was a young woman called Lois, who, Billington recounts, had suffered severe neurological impairment resulting from an accident during a stay in South Africa. The accident had severely affected the quality of Lois's life: she now experienced difficulties concentrating and, when under emotional strain, struggled to speak fluently. After a shared reading aloud of Frost's poem, Lois elaborated on the personal impact of her accident:

> A lot of my health problems started when I went to South Africa … but if I hadn't gone I would still probably be like: wanting to go here, want to go there. At the same time I wouldn't have the same … problems as I do now. Would I have the same mentality as now? Perhaps … something worse could have happened. Or I could have been worse if it had been easier.

Up until this point, Lois, Billington observes, 'tries not to make too much' of the accident, posing the kind of 'what-if' questions people are liable to ask themselves when mulling over life choices. But suddenly she changes tack:

> But if anyone was thinking of going and doing exploring … I'd say, don't do it, don't do this, don't do that, don't do the other … I'd be awful if if … I'd

be awful if if I ever had, if if I ever had, if if I ever, if ever had … children.
Because I'd be like, you're not doing that.

It's telling that Lois's sudden dysfluency pivots around the word 'if', a
conditional conjunction that conveys much of the regret and uncertainty at the
heart of the poem. It takes her several attempts to voice the final word of the
sentence: 'children'. What Lois knows, Billington observes, is that because of
her accident 'she is of course unlikely ever to have children … She has known
this, one might guess, for some time. But there are things one knows which one
cannot quite think.' And so the disclosure when it arrives, arrives obliquely: 'if
I ever had', where the word 'ever', Billington suggests, is likely to mean 'never.'

Lois's story is not so much voluntary as triggered. It is a moment of creative
inarticulacy, the difficult completion of a 'powerful sentence in a sensitive area',
with the poetry providing not only the atmosphere conducive to 'opening up
hidden lives' but also the language. The language of the poem, Billington argues,
provides for the release of what would otherwise be inexpressible or reduced
to platitude, a language that sparks 'inner echoes' – 'responses triggered and
inflected with the emotional vocabulary of the poem'.

In other (more expressly therapeutic) shared reading settings, Billington
shows how thinking through literary texts can be an effective means of
responding to physical and emotional issues, such as chronic pain and
depression. The higher demands that literature makes on readers, she argues,
produce 'closer concentration and absorbed attention', reducing awareness of
pain and distress – 'as though the extra mental effort' helps 'shift immersion
to another level'. Based on comparative studies of shared reading and
cognitive behavioural therapy (CBT), Billington claims that in some regards
literature-based interventions can be just as potent, if not more so, as standard
psychological management strategies.

In one comparative study, for example, Billington and colleagues found
that shared reading provided participants with 'better' thoughts about chronic

pain. Challenging negative thoughts and feelings is a vital part of managing persistent pain, the authors observe, and structured therapies like CBT help people overcome negative emotions by first recognizing and naming them. But during the CBT group sessions, the naming of emotions was top-down and explicit, typically conducted by the facilitators on behalf of the participants. In the shared reading groups, however, the naming of emotions was principally performed by readers themselves through the text, a far from passive process. A reading of Laurie Sheck's poem 'Mysteriously Standing', for instance, involved the participants interrogating rich metaphorical language in order to find new ways of interpreting and describing their condition. Here's the poem in full:

> All the fiercer and lawlessly irregular
> These intervals of withdrawal where I am a burned field
> And above me the sky is thickening and clouding.
> In that field, little Stonehenge of the heart
> Mysteriously standing, its distinct construction odd and uninjured in this yellow
> Light. If I say I was flexible, was harmed, was cleansed, was helped, was deeply marked,
> I still can't understand what I have been. Doubt falls in me falls through me
> A rough and intricate hazard. The mind carries an austere
> Inwardness that will not put out its eyes.

The phrases 'intervals of withdrawal where I am burned field' and 'little Stonehenge of the heart' proved particularly resonant to the participants, rendering their 'inner pain into articulacy':

> A: 'little Stonehenge' – it's like a kind of feeling that's been there for a long, long time.
> B: 'a burned field' – that's a really, really, *really* good way of describing yourself sometimes, isn't it?

Billington and her co-authors observe that B's response ('really, really, *really* good'), with its liveliness of manner and thought, is 'notably separate from the suffering she [B] recognizes and feels at another level'. Her response is 'a "good" thought (at once energetically vital and cognitively tolerable) *about* her own bad feelings – a thought which seems more descriptively accurate than she could have managed for herself, yet which does not feel imposed from without'.

But the poetry not only shifted personal perceptions of illness. The participants spoke of how the texts they read acted as a sustaining inner resource. The reading of poems such as Yeats's evocative 'The Lake Isle of Innisfree' had a transporting, meditative effect that endured for some time after the reading had finished. As one of the participants observed:

> From a poem or story, you get these pictures in your mind sometimes that you wouldn't normally get. You can sort of take them away … if you try to relax or when you go to bed of a night-time, you can have that picture in your mind that you got from the poem or story. What you have tried to absorb can come out later or help you as a distraction from all these things spinning round in your mind that you want to get rid of.

All told, shared reading had a prolonged and positive impact on chronic pain. The participants reported that both during and after the sessions their symptoms were less severe and they felt 'more fully themselves – more fulfilled and absorbed, more vitally alive'. Billington and colleagues are careful not to claim that shared reading is more effective than other interventions for chronic pain. But in demonstrating how reading and discussing literary texts help 'to recover a whole person, not just an ill one', they argue that shared reading can be a useful adjunct or longer-term follow-up to standard therapies.

The rise of bibliotherapy

Although shared reading responds to so much human strife and struggle, it would be wrong to see it as something solely for the sick and unhappy. The Reader's central mission is not to fix or heal people, but rather to promote the reading of serious books 'so that everyone can experience and enjoy great literature, which we believe is a tool for helping humans survive and live well'. Yet the rise of shared reading can be seen as part of, or at least coincides with, a broader trend of therapeutic reading, a growing interest in the use of books for ameliorative and restorative ends.

One doesn't have to look far for evidence of this bibliotherapeutic turn. Step into any high street bookstore and you'll find not only an ever-widening range of dedicated self-help titles but also bespoke collections of poems and stories (so-called poetic-pick-me-ups) designed to 'ease the mind' and 'nourish the soul', along with an increasing number of bibliomemoirs that celebrate the healing power of reading. If you're fed up with waiting to see a therapist, your doctor will likely be able to offer you a course of prescribed reading – an approved list of self-help texts that you can pick up from your local library. You don't even need a doctor's prescription: most public libraries have shelves devoted to 'mood-busting books', collections of non-fiction, fiction and poetry 'recommended by other readers to help lift your mood'. Outside of bookshops and libraries you can obtain therapeutic reading advice at a poetry pharmacy or bibliotherapy salon, or you can privately consult with one of a growing number of bibliotherapists who practise up and down the country. And nowadays many universities and colleges offer all manner of courses on bibliotherapy and reading for well-being. At Warwick University, for instance, you can take the 'world's first free online course devoted to the exploration of literature and mental health', a course that features exclusive interviews with luminaries such as Sir Ian McKellen, Melvyn Bragg, and Stephen Fry.

As this diverse range of activities suggests, bibliotherapy is a broad phenomenon that encompasses many different forms of reading for well-being. Although there now exists a well-established body of literature on the subject, there remains much debate in the field over what is, and what isn't, bibliotherapy, and how best to practise it. (Is it better suited to group or one-to-one settings? Should it be aimed at the healthy as well as the sick? Is it better to use fiction or non-fiction?) Nevertheless, most scholars and practitioners broadly agree on one thing: that the aim of bibliotherapy, whatever the method, is to guide people 'towards problem solving and coping in their personal lives'.

The term 'bibliotherapy' was coined and first used in print by the American essayist Samuel McChord Crothers in 1916. In a wonderfully whimsical essay, 'A Literary Clinic', published in *The Atlantic Monthly*, Crothers recounts a meeting with his friend the Reverend Augustus Bagster, who has recently set up a 'Bibliopathic Institute' at the church where he preaches. 'During the last year I have been working up a system of Biblio-therapeutics', Bagster tells Crothers. 'Bibliotherapy is … a new science', he explains. 'From my point of view, a book is a literary prescription put up for the benefit of some one who needs it.'

Bagster appears to have his bibliotherapeutic system all worked out, a book for every aspect of personal betterment: Ralph Waldo Emerson for 'wisdom', G. K. Chesterton for 'solid common sense', Jonathan Swift for 'acid truth'. The article ends when Bagster, to the author's disappointment, is abruptly summoned away by a client who has 'taken an overdose of war literature'. 'I was sorry,' writes Crothers, 'because I wished to discuss with him books which are at the same time stimulants and sedatives.'

Crothers describes bibliotherapy as a 'new science'. But the practice of recommending books for therapeutic ends is a time-honoured one, and one that remains at the heart of present-day bibliotherapy. Arguably the most well-established book prescribing scheme is the Reading Well Books on Prescription service, which operates in many British and American public libraries. The scheme was devised in 2003 by Professor Neil Frude, a clinical psychologist at the University of South Wales, who had the idea for the service when he was trying to figure out a way of making non-pharmacological treatments more accessible to his patients. At that time, the dominant mode of treating mental health problems was through drug intervention. But among doctors and patients there was, Frude writes, 'a growing awareness of the desirability of providing additional psychological therapies' to treat conditions such as depression and anxiety. Cognitive therapies such as CBT had been shown to be as effective as drug therapies, and since they promoted self-management skills, they were not only able to ameliorate patients' conditions but also help prevent future recurrences.

Since talking therapies were expensive and there were few suitably trained professionals available, Frude lit on the notion of using high-quality CBT self-help books, which were cheap to procure and readily accessible at local libraries. GPs could prescribe specific books for specific ailments, allowing patients to undertake step-by-step treatment programmes by themselves. A pilot was launched in Cardiff. It surpassed all expectations and was later rolled out to the rest of UK, quickly becoming the most widely adopted model of bibliotherapy in the country.

According to the website of The Reading Agency, a British charity that promotes reading and library use, 'over 2.6 million Reading Well books have been borrowed from [UK] libraries and 91% of people surveyed found their book helpful'. Many who completed the survey reported that their understanding of their mental health problem, as well as their confidence in managing it, had improved ... But for all the apparent success of the scheme, questions remain as to its overall impact on public health. Bibliotherapy, as Frude himself is quick to acknowledge, is not suitable for every kind of psychological ailment. 'As an "off-the-peg" treatment,' he writes, 'it would be inappropriate to use it with people who have severe conditions, those who are at high risk, or those whose problems are so complex or so atypical that no book could possibly address their condition.'

The effectiveness of the scheme, furthermore, very much depends on the dedication and commitment of those who use it. Self-help books and step-by-step programmes are not for everyone. The best sort of bibliotherapeutic help doesn't necessarily come from a dedicated self-help book. As the writer Blake Morrison puts it, 'Too often the prescribed "literature" in local libraries consists only of leaflets, or references to useful websites, or books written by "eminent therapists or former service users" which are worthy, practical-minded and dull. There's no recognition that people in trouble need more than the right labels.'

Unlike targeted self-help books, the use of imaginative literature offers an alternative, bottom-up approach to bibliotherapy. So-called 'creative bibliotherapy', which harnesses fiction, poetry, plays, and memoirs to enhance emotional well-being, places greater emphasis on the autonomy of the reader and their interaction with books. Here the experience of reading is just as important as the reading matter itself, which is not necessarily 'selected with specific therapeutic outcomes in mind' but is chosen for its 'relevance to the human condition'. There are many forms of creative bibliotherapy (group, one-to-one, self-directed, practitioner-led) and just as many underpinning psychological frameworks (person-centred, solution-focused, psychoanalytic). It is not always clear which supporting theory guides the action.

In their excellent book *Bibliotherapy*, Sarah McNicol and Liz Brewster argue that much of the therapeutic effect of creative bibliotherapy derives from three processes: identification, catharsis and insight. Identification, the first step, occurs when readers have an empathic response to a particular character or situation that reflects their own experience. To identify is to know that we are not alone, that our predicaments, our ways of being in the world, are not alienatingly unique. If readers sufficiently identify with a character or situation, they may experience catharsis – the release of, and relief from, pent-up tension and emotion. Catharsis is 'vicarious cleansing' – the purging of the audience's emotions through their representation in narrative and drama: readers share and immerse themselves in characters' situations and emotions, taking part in their journey and development. The final stage, insight, shifts the emphasis to the reader, who, having learned through the experiences of a particular character, applies the character's situation to their own life.

This three-step approach underpins bibliotherapy interventions in a range of clinical and community settings. The literature abounds with examples of readers experiencing catharsis and insight, an internal change helped along by professional facilitators. In one of my favourite studies, the psychotherapist Cristina Martins, who practises bibliotherapy in an addiction rehabilitation centre for young people, describes the cathartic effect that reading and discussing poetry has had on her patients. Most of her young (fifteen- to thirty-five-year-old) clients, Martins relates, come from impoverished backgrounds, where they have had little contact with books, and what experience they have had of reading has 'left them with feelings of frustration or impotence towards the written culture'.

But in a group setting, books come alive for these young people, become, as it were, partners in thought, helping them to reevaluate their lives and conceive a better future. In one particularly illustrative session, a patient asked to read the poem 'Last Song' by the Spanish poet Miguel Hernández, the first verse of which reads:

Painted, not void:
my house is painted
with the vast colour
of tragedy and passion.

Martins points out that patients with substance use disorders are often unable to throw off the shackles of the present: 'they feel disconnected from their past and unable to project themselves into the future'. The present they inhabit, is a very narrow, constricting one: 'everyday life revolves around getting the substance, consuming it, suffering its absence and regaining strength to re-consume'. Yet in the group discussion following the reading, the patients, through the agency of the poem and the promptings of the therapist, were able to articulate their past and future situations, thereby confronting the 'tyranny' of the present:

A: It [the poem] made me remember my grandmother's house ... It was a very neat house and very clean. There was always a smell of delicious food because my grandmother always cooked ... nobody made custard like her ... She died a few years ago ... she was like my mother ... more than a mother ... she was always there.

D: It made me think that I don't have a house: I live on the street; I sleep in a night hostel ... at my age it's a failure.

A: Noooo, why? There are stages of life. You are going to have your own house yet.

In short, the bibliotherapy sessions helped Martins's patients to project themselves into the future – to imagine a new life for themselves. Reading and discussing poetry with others, moreover, provided them with a private sanctuary, a shelter from their current adversities, reducing, in turn, their levels of anxiety and the urge to use substances again.

***

Martins's reading intervention is undeniably impressive. But equally striking are those cases of bibliotherapy where readers find their own way to recovery. One of the most celebrated cases of personal recovery through reading in the annals of bibliotherapy is that of John Stuart Mill, the English philosopher and political economist.

Mill was one of the most famous child prodigies in history, rigorously schooled in Benthamite philosophy by his father James Mill, a dour and exacting taskmaster (he had his son learn Greek and arithmetic at the age of three). Under the influence of his father's utilitarian world view, the young Mill believed that success in life rested on his being a true 'reformer of the world', a project which he pursued with unremitting fervour. In the autumn of 1826, however, Mill experienced a profound crisis in his mental history and sank into a deep depression. His work suddenly had no meaning or relevance to him; nothing interested him anymore, such that, as he put it in his autobiography, he 'seemed to have nothing left to live for'.

What deepened Mill's despair was that he had no-one to turn to. His father would have been his natural recourse, but Mill senior, a cold and imposing figure, was the last person he could turn to for help. He would have no insight into his son's mental state, and even if he had, 'he was,' Mill wrote, 'not the physician who could heal it'. Nor was there relief for the young Mill in his favourite books – 'those memorials of past nobleness and greatness' from which he 'had always hitherto drawn strength and animation'. He read them now without conviction or feeling, becoming increasingly persuaded that his love for humanity had 'worn itself out'.

Nevertheless, it was a book that saved Mill. In the autumn of 1828, out of curiosity and with no expectation of relief, he took up a collection of Wordsworth's poems. He wasn't customarily inclined to poetry. ('Quantity of pleasure being equal, pushpin is as good as poetry' ran the famous Benthamite dictum.) His mind, by his own account, had become 'irretrievably analytic' – his ability to feel eroded by all that Gradgrind utilitarian instruction. But Wordsworth was a revelation. Precisely what he needed:

> What made Wordsworth's poems a medicine for my state of mind, was that they expressed, not mere outward beauty, but states of feeling, and of thought coloured by feeling, under the excitement of beauty. They seemed to be the very culture of feelings, which I was in quest of. In them I seemed to draw from a source of inward joy, of sympathetic and imaginative pleasure, which could be shared in by all human beings, which had no

connexion with struggle or imperfection, but would be made richer by every improvement in the physical or social condition of mankind. From them I seemed to learn what would be the perennial sources of happiness, when all the greater evils of life shall have been removed. And I felt myself at once better and happier as I came under their influence.

From Wordsworth Mill learned not only how to escape his despair, but that he was not alone in suffering it. For he discovered that the poet had had a similar experience to his own, that he too 'had felt that the first freshness of youthful enjoyment of life was not lasting; but that he had sought for compensation, and found it, in the way in which he was now teaching me to find it'.

Mill slowly, but steadily, emerged from his depression, and never suffered a relapse. He went on to write several highly influential books of philosophy, economics and history, and became the leading liberal philosopher of his generation. Throughout his life, he continued to read and appreciate Wordsworth's poetry. There were greater poets, he writes, than Wordsworth, but

poetry of deeper and loftier feeling could not have done for me at that time what his did. I needed to be made to feel that there was real, permanent happiness in tranquil contemplation. Wordsworth taught me this, not only without turning away from, but with a greatly increased interest in the common feelings and common destiny of human beings.

Fiction prescriptions

Poetry worked for Mill. But it doesn't work for everyone. Many bibliotherapists believe that fiction is the supreme healer. In their best-selling book, *The Novel Cure: An A-Z of Literary Remedies*, Ella Berthoud and Susan Elderkin claim that novels and short stories are 'the purest and best form of bibliotherapy'.

It's a claim they base on their own experience of working with 'patients' – 'bolstered', as they put it, by a wealth of anecdotal evidence.

> Sometimes it's the story that charms; sometimes it's the rhythm of the prose that works on the psyche, stilling or stimulating. Sometimes it's an idea or an attitude suggested by a character in a similar quandary or jam. Either way, novels have the power to transport you into another existence, and see the world from a different point of view.

The Novel Cure is premised on the idea that fiction can handle most things that life can throw at us. And some more. Taking the form of a medical dictionary, the book offers remedies not only for common problems (for depression try Slyvia Plath's *The Bell Jar*, for anxiety Henry James's *The Portrait of a Lady*) but also for lesser-known ailments such as 'itchy teeth' (Saul Bellow: *Henderson the Rain King*) and 'fear of dinner parties' (Ali Smith: *There but for the*). The authors even venture a cure for constipation in the form of Gregory David Roberts's novel *Shantaram*: 'Read it', they suggest, 'for the ease with which the words tumble out'. Literary fiction, it appears, works just as well on the bowels as it does on the mind.

These sillier 'cures' aside, many of the recommendations in *The Novel Cure* are seemingly sensible ones. For those dealing with grief, Berthoud and Elderkin recommend John Berger's consoling *Here Is Where We Meet* (a revelation to me). For readers struggling to come to terms with failure, they suggest H. G. Wells's *The History of Mr Polly*: 'Our guess is that, by the end, your sense of the inevitability of failure for yourself and Mr Polly, will have absquatulated into thin air.' (Though to my mind, the most consoling book about failure is Joe Moran's *If You Should Fail*, a book, incidentally, that happens to be a work of non-fiction. This is one of the appeals of *The Novel Cure*, 'the way it drives you to agree or disagree with the authors' choices'.)

For all its useful recommendations, however, it's difficult to say whether *The Novel Cure* has any 'real healing power for readers'. As the doctor and writer Gavin Francis points out, the book 'does not distinguish between emotional and physical pain' such that one finds remedies for broken bones as well as broken hearts. But no work of literature can shrink a tumour or mend a fracture (and in fairness the authors do not claim that it can: their reading suggestion for a broken leg – *Cleave* by Nikki Gemmell – pivots around the idea of keeping the reader sane during the long period of convalescence rather than the author's 'inventive prose' knitting the bone back together). *The Novel Cure* is more of a bibliophile's billet-doux than a serious work of bibliotherapy, 'an exuberant pageant of literary fiction and a celebration of the possibilities of the novel'. It's a book that works best, Francis suggests, when it tackles perennial existential issues – fear, loss, loneliness – rather than specific clinical complaints.

Berthoud and Elderkin have been prescribing books to patients since 2008, when they set up a bibliotherapy service at Alain de Botton's The School of Life in central London. They offer one-to-one in-person and remote consultations, at the end of which clients receive a personalized reading prescription designed to 'open up new perspectives' and 're-enchant the world'. Before their consultation, clients fill out a questionnaire that asks them about their reading habits and well-being. ('Did books feature largely in your childhood?' 'Do you always finish the books you start?' 'What is preoccupying you at the moment?' 'What is missing from your life?' And so on.)

When the novelist Ceridwen Dovey consulted with Berthoud – an experience she elegantly describes in the New Yorker – she found herself surprised by what she 'wanted to confess' to the bibliotherapist. 'I am worried,' she wrote, 'about having no spiritual resources to shore myself up against the inevitable future grief of losing somebody I love … I'm not religious, and I don't particularly want to be, but I'd like to read more about other people's reflections on coming to some sort of early, weird form of faith in a "higher being" as an emotional survival tactic.'

When I had my own bibliotherapy session with Berthoud, my troubles seemed rather trivial at the side of Dovey's pressing existential quandaries (my cardinal concerns were to hit me a few years later). When Berthoud asked what was bothering me, the only thing that came to mind was the book I was struggling to write. I kept putting it off, I told her, was worried that I'd never finish the thing and that even if I did, it wouldn't be anything like the book I'd been contracted to write. (She made a swift suggestion: Dodie Smith's *I Capture the Castle*. It will 'help you unblock your writing mind, being a brilliant spur to the joys of writing, as well as showing an unusual way of catalyzing a writer into doing their job.')

If truth be told, I hadn't expected much from the consultation: I thought it'd be little more than an interesting, if slightly expensive, chat about books with a very pleasant person. But when one talks about books one inevitably gives oneself away, and I found myself excitedly talking about things I wouldn't otherwise have talked about, or at least talked about so openly – viz. my struggle to read when I was younger, how as a child I couldn't get into books, just didn't have the patience or attention span for them – they felt like work, a slog, something to be got through – my parents knew the stakes and did their best (ours was not a bookish house), but I was immune to the charm of words, the patent delight of rhyme and story, and I left school at sixteen (with three GCSEs) and went to work on a building site – my love of reading came later, I told Berthoud, after I had joined the police service and chanced upon the poetry of Philip Larkin, whose work I first encountered when I was pursuing a shoplifter, the two of us, pursuer and pursued, having ended up in the book section of WHSmith, where, to maintain my cover, I picked up the closest book to hand – it was the *Collected Poems* – and it completely blew me away – I thought poetry was all about larks and daffodils, not stubbing one's fags out on saucer-souvenir trays, or watching light move, or waves folding behind villages (such meticulous noticings! such concealed imaginings!) – and I read most of the book in one standing (yes, yes, he got away – but I got my Larkin!), and I knew then and there that something had unlocked within me, that my life would be, must be somewhere else, that from now on I would see the world in a different way.

A few days after my session with Berthoud, my reading prescription arrived. It was a wide-ranging, enticing list – *The Year of the Hare* by Arto Paasalinna, *Cosmicomics* by Italo Calvino, *The Last Samurai* by Helen DeWitt, among others – and I set about it dutifully, beginning with the Paasalinna. But no sooner had I started the book than I abandoned it in favour of the next one on the list, which in turn I abandoned in favour of the one after that, and so on and on, each successive title having somehow the greater claim on my attention than its predecessor. No matter how hard I tried, I just couldn't work my way through the list, and by way of displacement began working on my book again.

Ceridwen Dovey, however, savoured her fiction prescription. Over the course of several years, she read every one of Berthoud's recommendations (a similarly varied list that included Herman Hesse's *Siddhartha* and Saul Bellow's *Henderson the Rain King*). Although during the course of her prescribed reading she was fortunate enough to have her 'ability to withstand terrible grief untested', the books helped her through an unrelated difficulty: an unexpected bout of 'acute physical pain' from which she suffered for several months. She wasn't exactly sure how the reading helped with the pain. The insights gleaned from the books, she writes, 'are still nebulous, as learning gained through reading fiction often is – but therein lies its power'. As she explains:

> In a secular age, I suspect that reading fiction is one of the few remaining paths to transcendence, that elusive state in which the distance between the self and the universe shrinks. Reading fiction makes me lose all sense of self, but at the same time makes me feel most uniquely myself. As Woolf, the most fervent of readers, wrote, a book 'splits us into two parts as we read', for 'the state of reading consists in the complete elimination of the ego', while promising 'perpetual union' with another mind.

Dissensions

At the end of my bibliotherapy session, I asked Berthoud whether she thought prescribing fiction risked medicalizing reading, reducing works of literature to little more than functional self-help texts.

'That was something we were accused of when *The Novel Cure* first came out,' she said. 'Yes, there is that danger, and we very much try to avoid that sense of treating books like they're purely a curative device. We're very conscious that literature is all about art, beauty, lyricism, language … We really want to avoid that feeling of treating books like they're just a medicine.'

Nevertheless, the charge of medicalization persists. One of the most prominent and eloquent critics of bibliotherapy is the literary scholar Leah Price, who, in a series of wryly perceptive books and articles, challenges the belief that reading novels is unequivocally good for you. For Price, bibliotherapy initiatives raise 'troubling questions' about the value of reading. 'What's lost,' she asks, 'when a bookshelf is repurposed as a medicine cabinet – and when a therapist's job gets outsourced to the page?' Reading, she argues, has been pressed into 'the service of mental and physical wellbeing', such that hurtling through a book 'to find out what happens next, seeing the world through a character's eyes, wallowing in the play of language' has become a means to a clinical end. 'Today, for an increasing number of people, the pleasures of reading require a doctor's note.'

But what troubles Price most of all is the way that bibliotherapy has encroached on other disciplines, especially her own, that of literary criticism. The rise of bibliotherapy, it seems, has brought about a kind of turf war between literary experts (academic critics) and literary amateurs (bibliotherapists and other practitioners who work with literary texts). As part of their 'project of making literature more usable to lay readers', bibliotherapists risk, Price argues, 'making literary criticism less so'. She sees bibliotherapy not only as a threat to the function and authority of literary criticism but also to the critical thinking that criticism fosters: 'instead of inciting readers to rage (as a critic might have done a generation ago) against the patriarchal logic of the sonnet, a bibliotherapy course at University of Warwick instead uses poems to "calm" and "reassure" readers. What's therapeutic here is the reading of literature – but not literary reading'.

That's well put. But I'm not so sure that literary reading and therapeutic reading are mutually exclusive (shared reading, which involves carefully examining 'the turns and nuances and telling details' of a text, is surely a form of literary reading, a form of close, immersive reading). But Price is right to question the ever-expanding realm of bibliotherapy, not least the roll-out of the Books on Prescription scheme in lieu of proper funding for public services. 'A public library system suffering even more drastic budget cuts than the health service,' she observes, 'was in no position to turn away the foot traffic, funding, and legitimacy that Book Prescription supplied.'

All the same, I think it's fair to say that Price has little good to say about bibliotherapy. There's little concession that it might play a part in healing or otherwise help people live their lives. Literature, it seems, is perhaps better off in the seminar room, read solely on its own terms, literature qua literature. (Derek Attridge: literature 'solves no problems and saves no souls'. But what's literature for if it's not for thinking and feeling with, for doing with?)

Another, more urgent, question that hangs over bibliotherapy is simply: does it work? Throughout its history bibliotherapy has been criticized for its lack of methodological and quantitative rigour. The evidence underpinning many bibliotherapy studies takes the form of small data sets from which findings cannot readily be generalized or extrapolated, and much of the research literature promoting bibliotherapy tends to be confined to niche publications or, as Raymond Tallis less charitably puts it, 'fourth-rate journals'.

Over the last few decades, however, there has been more quantitative evaluation of bibliotherapy schemes, with researchers adopting the 'gold-standard' meta-analytic approach (a statistical evaluation of multiple independent studies). Such meta-analysis studies have shown that non-fiction bibliotherapy is effective at responding to mild-to-moderate anxiety and depression, along with other specific conditions such as panic disorder and alcohol dependency. Books, according to these large-scale meta-analytic studies, don't outperform professional therapists – and not everyone who engages with self-help literature improves after treatment – but bibliotherapy can still be considered effective, these studies conclude, since disorders like anxiety tend not to abate without treatment.

The quantitative picture for creative bibliotherapy is less clear. As these pages have shown, much of the supporting evidence for literature-based interventions is derived from personal testimonies, anecdotes, and observations, all of which are susceptible to interpretive bias and subjective validation. On the face of it, however, the evidence is promising, with studies showing that creative bibliotherapy and shared reading can help reduce the symptoms of mood and anxiety disorders and promote well-being. More quantitative measures such as controlled trials and surveys are needed, critics argue, to empirically assess the therapeutic power of literary texts. But at the very least, the available evidence indicates that creative bibliotherapy can serve as an effective adjunct to more traditional treatments, as well as helping people who might not otherwise seek or receive therapy.

And yet, as much as further quantitative research would strengthen its evidence base, evaluating bibliotherapy in strictly positivist terms risks failing to capture the subtleties and complexities of people's experiences of reading, which vary from reader to reader. The kinds of emotive, aesthetic texts (fiction, poetry, plays) used in creative bibliotherapy and shared reading interventions, and the subjective language readers use to describe them, are incommensurate with scientific objectivity. Quantitative instruments have their place, but they tell us little about how books make an impression on us or how they change our lives.

These methodological issues are unlikely to be resolved anytime soon. In the end, I suspect that bibliotherapists 'may never be able to capture' the kind and quantity of data that 'scientists hunger for', that is, the kind of data that sways the opinions of funders and policy makers. But that still leaves us with the personal testimony of countless readers down the centuries, a living and ever-expanding database that, as Jonathan Bate and Andrew Schuman remind us, 'speaks volumes for those who care to listen'.

2

What have libraries ever done for us? In defence of the public library system

If she did not make a point of getting herself out to the shops and to the library … it would be possible to go for weeks without seeing anyone.

– ALISON MOORE

You rarely see a police officer in the library …

– ERIC KLINENBERG

1

On 18 December 2014, the British government published the Sieghart report, an independent review on the future of public libraries, led by the publisher and entrepreneur William Sieghart. Public library reviews are common and invariably come to nothing, but the Sieghart review promised to be something different. Commissioned by the Department for Culture, Media and Sport, it had been eagerly anticipated by librarians, booksellers and publishers, who saw it as the report which, unlike its many predecessors, could bring about real change to the public library system, revitalizing and securing its future.

The government, in the voice of Edward Vaizey, the then Minister of State for Culture, Communications and Creative Industries, ostensibly welcomed the report, promising to implement its key recommendations, in the first instance setting up a task force to begin the process, but conveniently failed to comment on the shortfalls in library funding to which the report had alluded. Vaizey rounded off his brief communique by describing the public library service as a 'cherished part of our cultural heritage, and a key player for the future', remarks that rang rather hollow given that his austerity government had presided over the biggest programme of library closures in British history.

Not long after the release of the Sieghart review, I paid a visit to Angel Row library in Nottingham city centre. The library had been my stomping ground when I worked as a police officer in the 1990s, and returning to the old place was something of a homecoming for me, a return to my intellectual roots. The library had served as a bolthole at an uncertain point in my life, a place where I'd spent many a happy, self-improving hour immersed in the stacks (all part of my grand scheme of trying to figure out what to do with my life). In the quiet seclusion of the library, safely out of sight of the sergeant and inspector, I was able to pursue my autodidactic impulses with impunity, free to hatch my secret plan of escape. (None of my colleagues, I'm sure of it, ever suspected that I was leading a kind of double life.)

At that time, I had near-licence to roam the city during my working hours. I was temporarily attached to a retail crime unit, a secondment that mainly involved the mindless routine of processing (interviewing, fingerprinting) shoplifters. It was relentless work, particularly during the busy shopping days when the stores fielded extra security staff, but during the quieter parts of the week there was often little to do besides catch up on paperwork, and the time was effectively your own. Some of my colleagues would occupy themselves by running errands that took them dubiously out of the city, but I spent the time scouring the streets for seasoned shop thieves, who, with their bulky foil-lined carrier bags (for going equipped to steal), stood out easily enough among the crowds of shoppers and office workers.

At first I relished this undercover work, found it thrilling in a *Boys' Own* kind of way. I would select a likely looking suspect and then, like the narrator of Edgar Allan Poe's story 'The Man of the Crowd', resolve 'to follow the stranger whithersoever he would go'. Yet for all the intrigue and excitement of the pursuit, I had no desire to actually confront whoever I was tailing. It was more the idea of doing so that appealed to me – I was indulging in a time-wasting fantasy, an elaborate exercise in escape and distraction, and after a while I abandoned these notional pursuits altogether in favour of simply wandering about the city, walking without object or purpose.

The walks became increasingly protracted, sometimes taking me miles away from the police station. On these longer excursions I felt little compulsion to head back at the end of the shift and would continue maundering aimlessly, as if in a Sebaldian fugue, hoping in some vague way that I might lose myself (in all senses of the phrase) in ever secluded parts of the city. Partly out of boredom, partly to satisfy some indeterminate but insistent inner need, I found myself drifting towards book shops and the public library. At that time there were still lots of bookstores operating in the city centre (numerous branches of Dillons, Blackwell's, WHSmith, along with the wonderfully sepulchral Jermy & Westerman on Mansfield Road), each of which offered new worlds of possibility. Yet despite some enjoyable hours nosing about their stacks, I was never quite able to settle myself in book shops. There was only so much time you could comfortably squander in them without spending money (Jermy & Westerman excepted), and after a while I began to feel increasingly self-conscious, felt that the staff had me down as some sort of ne'er-do-well, someone dubiously killing time, waiting for something else. Which, of course, I was.

By contrast, I felt at ease in the public library. I was not a library lover by inclination, had always felt, in the words of Alberto Manguel, that 'the love of libraries, like other loves, must be learnt'. Libraries had always seemed to me to be exclusive and faintly intimidating places – there was a whiff of the quasi-religious about them, something oppressively sedate. But Angel Row was unlike other libraries I recalled visiting in my youth. It was the first library I'd used that approximated to what William Gass calls a 'great library', that is, a library of 'density' and 'scope', a library whose holdings are so extensive that 'no one quite knows what is in its basements'. Although I was a fledgling serious reader, acutely aware of how few books I'd read, and how little I knew, the endless, where-does-one-begin? rows of books presented themselves less as an accusation than as an invitation, an opportunity to enrich myself on my own terms and at my own fickle rate. This seemingly infinite supply of reading (I believed the library contained the whole of world literature) offered a way of working out some new direction and, as vague as it sounds, resolving something – whatever it was – within me.

Not only was Angel Row a library of scope and density, but it was also welcoming (another of Gass's key criteria). The place accommodated you no matter who you were or what your purpose, or lack of purpose: I spent a fair amount of time simply relishing being alone among other people, who also wanted to be alone among other people. I soon established a comfortable routine for myself, occupying a table on the third floor – my long shanks stretched out beneath it – that was within easy reach of stacks of essays, poetry, plays, philosophy and fiction, all of which were unfamiliar to me but in which I discovered kindred sensibilities, as well as new ways of perceiving and responding to the world. Since I was merely following some nebulous instinct, I read in a desultory and half-knowing way, taking down books and opening them up at random. There was absolutely nothing scholarly about the process (scholarliness came later). And yet, more by blundering persistence than anything else, I came to realize that what I was doing was increasingly important to me, that I had to keep on asking questions, to keep on turning the pages.

All told, I spent two years escaping to Angel Row. After my secondment ended, I returned to frontline policing, where the constraints of shiftwork curtailed my sorties to the library. But by then it didn't matter. Angel Row had afforded me a glimpse of another country, the tantalizing prospect of exchanging one life for another. It was only a matter of time (another two years joylessly working the beat) before I left the service and eventually secured a place at university, after which, as they say, I never looked back. Indeed, writing about it now, it's strange to think that police work ever appealed to me, and that I served, or rather survived, in the force for as long (eight years) as I did.

***

Although I craved a spot of nostalgia, wanted to recover something of the past, my return trip to Angel Row was not solely an exercise in sentimentality. A few days before my visit, I'd been reading (in the name of research, I hasten to add) the online diary of John Redwood. In one particularly sniffy entry, the Tory MP described a visit he'd made to an unspecified public library. 'During the half hour I was in or near it,' he wrote, 'I did not see anyone borrow a book … There were not that many books on offer. It was predominantly a fiction library. The crime section seemed to be the single biggest themed area.' The non-fiction offer proved equally unappealing: 'The books seemed oriented to middle class hobbies like antiques and foreign travel. I guess the book buying had been well judged to cater for the demand of a fairly affluent local community.' In short it seemed that the library 'was not worth stopping for'.

Such an uninspiring visit only served to reinforce Redwood's belief that the public library, far from being an equalizer, was more an outfit tailored to satisfy the needs of the middle classes than those of the wider community. In an era of what he referred to as 'tighter spending controls', it was therefore only right, he argued, that 'we need to think again how many libraries we need in each community'.

It seemed to me that, even before he set foot in the library, Redwood had made up his mind about the place. He certainly had nothing good to say about it. But of course a fleeting half-hour visit, during which no attempt was made to speak to library staff or patrons, can hardly be said to constitute a thorough assessment. I wanted to go off on my own Redwoodian escapade, to see for myself whether the public library had become little more than a book borrowing service for the bourgeoisie. Redwood's provocation aside, I also wanted to know how the public library was faring in times of austerity, to assess the impact of funding reductions on provision. As libraries were closing up and down the country, government ministers euphemistically spoke of 'fiscal responsibility' and 'difficult decisions', language that glossed over the very real effects that spending cuts were having on people's lives.

It was an apt time to return to and appraise Angel Row, Nottingham's largest, principal library. Nottingham City Council, in response to funding shortfalls, had recently undertaken a participatory budgeting exercise, a kind of civic version of 'I'm a Celebrity... Get Me Out of Here!', in which the local community were gamely invited to rate the quality of its public services – taking part entered you into a free prize draw to win tickets to the local pantomime (*Aladdin* that year) – and help determine where the axe should fall. Much as I saw this as a face-saving attempt at relieving the local authority of the burden of difficult financial decision-making, I had sympathy for the Council, whose cut of funding from central government, compared to many other (much more affluent) authorities, was disproportionately high. Having had its overall spending power reduced by close on £70 million (5.5%) since 2013, the Council was now facing unprecedented budgetary challenges and having to make significant savings, which would inevitably involve some degree of service reduction.

As the spate of library closures across the country had demonstrated, libraries were deemed to be soft targets and hence one of the first public services to be cut. The crude logic that informed such decision-making was perhaps best exemplified in comments made by the former Mayor of Doncaster, Peter

Davies, who, against considerable public opposition, had implemented a number of cuts to the region's libraries. To close a library, he conceded, was 'unfortunate', but to shut down a care home was 'totally unacceptable'. (Who would've thought keeping a library open necessarily entailed closing down a care home?) But my favourite vindication came from Keith Mitchell, Leader of Oxford County Council, who framed the argument in similarly Manichean, yet even more outlandish, terms: 'to exempt libraries from cuts is a call to heap more cuts on the elderly, learning disabled and those with mental health problems. Have they [the library campaigners] thought through the impact of their messianic message about literature on the most vulnerable in our society?'

In these and kindred arguments there was little recognition, let alone appreciation, of what libraries actually contribute to the public good (including their contribution to health and social inclusion). Libraries were deemed to be a financial liability, a burden on other services. They were dispensable – their closure an unquestionable necessity.

2

Angel Row Library is housed in a five-storey Victorian building whose façade, despite its automatic doors and corporate lime-green livery, still has something of a nineteenth-century municipal feel about it. The building bears little trace of its former commercial incarnation – the furniture store, Henry Baker Smart & Brown – which traded here, up until 1974, for just under 100 years. Although the library is cherished by staff and users alike, the building itself is held in no great affection. Costly and difficult to maintain, it has long been in a state of poor repair, sporting many of the same signs of wear and tear – gum-flecked carpet tiles, cracked paint and peeling wallpaper – with which I'd been familiar twenty years ago. Nonetheless, surrounded by endlessly proliferating fast-food outlets and high street chains, the building has the virtue of being the only 'structural reminder of civic values' in an area now exclusively given over to commerce and consumption.

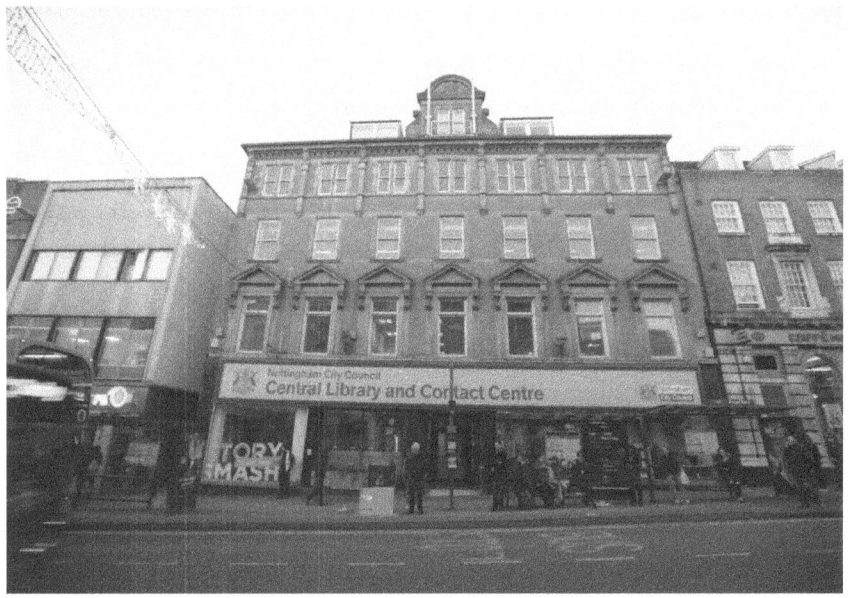

Directly in front of the library is a series of busy bus stops. I remembered how, years ago, approaching the entrance to the place often felt like running the gauntlet, how edging through the bustle of passengers and pedestrians only served, as you left the street, to emphasize the relative tranquillity of the building's interior. When you enter the library nowadays, you are no longer greeted by welcoming quiet. Instead, you step into a lively scene of harried counter staff and petitioning queues – queues petitioning not for books but for benefits and housing advice. In the intervening years, the ground floor had been repurposed to include a joint services centre that provided benefit and housing services – services which were formerly located in various buildings around the city centre but which the Council had sold off to private developers. Having all these services under one roof was no doubt cost-effective and convenient for the Council, but this restructuring, as the lively scene before me testified, had affected the library environment, imparting something of an institutional edge to it, an impression reinforced by the presence of two security guards who stood about the lobby (looking this morning, however, not so much imposing and official, as shiftless and bored).

Outside of the service centre waiting area, the remainder of the ground floor was still library territory – space dedicated to books and the reading of books. Part of the pleasure of browsing the shelves here had been encountering obscure, out-of-print books – T. F. Powy's *God's Eyes A-Twinkle*, Denton Welch's *A Voice Through A Cloud* – works of fiction long fallen out of literary favour. And so it was heartening to see that there was still an eclectic range of titles on display, spanning popular fiction to mainstream and lesser-known classics. Although there was a considerable amount of genre fiction – crime especially (heaven forfend!) – there were also numerous independent titles: for every Hachette and HarperCollins, there was a Salt and Serpent's Tail nearby. It was no surprise – though no less of a pleasant discovery – to come across Alison Moore's *The Pre-War House and Other Stories*, a book which I'd long been looking out for, but never encountered, in my local Waterstones.

As I popped to the counter with my Alison Moore, wondering all the while what John Redwood would have made of the book stock here, I caught sight of another new development: the presence of self-service points. There were several of these units scattered about the library, but no one appeared to be using them (which pleased me). I'm not a luddite by any means – I recognize the benefits of self-service kiosks: convenience and anonymity, theoretical speed and efficiency – but all the same I found their presence dispiriting. The roll-out of self-service provision was an index of the growing de-professionalization of the library workforce. Where once staff issued books and other items to patrons, now library users, momentarily pitched into the labour process, do the job for themselves. Although the public are not obliged to use these self-service points, they are very much encouraged to: brightly illuminated and prominently positioned, the machines clamour for one's attention, their inescapability testament to the fact that staff are expected to push up to 95% of transactions through them.

Here and elsewhere, the library was busy. In the main study areas on the upper floors, virtually all the tables were occupied, including, I noticed with a pang of envy, my old desk, at which sat Tom, books stacked on either side of him like tottering columns of poker chips. Tom, who was studying for his A levels (Theatre Studies today), told me that he preferred working in the public library to working at home or school, where there were 'too many distractions and not enough books'. He described himself as a relatively new user of the library, having only recently discovered a more suitable place to study. 'There aren't many tables in the school library,' he said, 'and the atmosphere is better here. I like being among other people. It encourages you to work.'

Sitting across from Tom was Aziz, who was poring over a copy of the *Jang*, an Urdu newspaper, which was spread out, recto and verso, before him. He'd just returned from a trip to Mecca. 'It was warmer there, but I was missing the paper!' A user of the library for seven years ('ever since I retired'), he told me that he enjoyed being here ('just sitting and relaxing'), liked the peace and the presence of others. 'It's not the same reading the paper at home. Home is home, you know, but here you meet other people. Can talk if you want.'

Leaving Tom and Aziz to reconnect to the civic current, I returned to the ground floor, where snuggled in a den-like corner at the far end of the room, library staff were reading nursery rhymes aloud with young children. This was Totstime, a lively music and storytelling group for the under-fives and their parents. Totstime was a 'godsend' for Tara, who, plumped down in soft cushions with her four-year-old son Jack, told me that although she read to him as often as she could at home, it was a challenge to maintain his interest, to make him feel comfortable with books and stories. Coming to the library was a way of getting him excited about reading, making it fun and more accessible. 'I want to introduce him to songs and nursery rhymes, to keep him interested,' she said. 'But it's not easy by yourself. I want to encourage him, and being here among other people helps me do that.'

The wonderful thing about activities such as Totstime is that not only are they great fun (I defy even the most moveless of souls to resist joining in with a communal singing of 'Miss Polly had a Dolly'), but they also confer, as Jack and Tara's experiences attest, many social and developmental benefits, enhancing children's early literacy and supporting relationships with parents. In such a collaborative context, the communal singing of nursery rhymes and songs heightens children's sensitivity to language, delightfully disguising the fact that they are being exposed to complex literacy conventions such as grammar and syntax (think of 'The House that Jack Built' with its endless string of relative clauses: 'This is the cat, that killed the rat, that ate the malt …'), the acquisition of which is vital for linguistic development. Given Nottingham's relatively poor rates of child literacy, Totstime was a timely activity ('intervention' is too clinical, too joyless a word), providing parents who might struggle with reading the chance to directly involve themselves in their children's education.

Sadly, however, the value and popularity of groups such as Totstime had not made them any less vulnerable to the effects of budgetary constraints. 'The cuts have forced us to be creative,' one of the senior librarians told me. 'We can't do what we've always done. We've really had to change our offer – do more with less money.' Doing 'more with less' had inevitably resulted in the library having to curtail a number of its activities – not just inessential provision, but services that had had a real effect on people's lives.

One such service was The Big Book Share, a project which aimed, through the sharing of read-aloud stories, to bring together parents in prison with their children outside. The scheme, a collaboration between HMP Nottingham and Nottingham City Libraries, involved prisoners reading stories onto a compact disc for their children to listen to at home. Although well-intentioned prison projects 'can sometimes have a whiff of do-goodery about them', as Terence Blacker puts it, The Big Book Share scheme had yielded impressive results, strengthening families by enabling parents to contribute to their children's reading development (as Blacker points out, stories are neutral: when prisoners read to their children they are afforded 'an element of normality', the chance to feel like parents again).

Besides delight and connection through storytelling, at the heart of schemes such as The Big Book Share and Totstime is the well-attested idea that parental involvement is positively related to children's educational performance. Simply put, the children of parents who regularly engage in reading (regardless of their occupational status) are more likely to have higher literacy levels. But providing dedicated literacy support for families relies on the expertise of trained librarians whose work in child literacy cannot easily, if at all, be undertaken by volunteers who are increasingly taking over the running of libraries.

'There's no doubt we're a vulnerable service now,' the librarian told me. 'People who use us love us. But our survival isn't a given any longer.'

3

Was there ever a golden age of the public library? I'd always assumed that libraries, like parks, museums and town halls, were places that had been, and would forever be, part of the fabric of civic life. But the political and economic foundations on which public libraries were built and sustained have always been parlous.

Right from the beginning, prior to the Public Libraries Act of 1850, which brought about the public library system, there was little political appetite for a free book lending service levied by taxation. Library provision back then was patchy across Britain, with facilities in the main provided by conscience-stricken philanthropists concerned with educating the industrial working class. With the passing of the Public Libraries Act, however, the right of every town to have a free public library was established. The bill had a difficult journey through parliament, which at that time was mainly made up of MPs from the propertied classes who saw no economic benefit in having a free public library service. Libraries were non-profit-making and, worst still, potential hotbeds of sedition, places which 'might give rise to an unhealthy agitation'. Even later in the nineteenth century, when the public library had become more of a community landmark, it continued to be seen as a kind of 'socialists' continuation school', a den of idle diversion. As one scandalized commentator put it at the time: 'Free Libraries are "god-sends" to the town loafer, who finds himself housed and amused at the public expense, and may lounge away his time among the intellectual luxuries which his neighbours are taxed to provide for him.'

But for all the reactionary clamour of the ruling classes, the public library continued to grow briskly, and by the beginning of the twentieth century a national library service could be said to have taken discernible, if tentative, shape. Public expenditure on libraries remained low, and the development of existing services owed more to the charitable donations of private benefactors, such as Andrew Carnegie, the self-made steel magnet, than the investment of local authorities. 'There are few doors which a golden key will not unlock,' Carnegie pronounced at the opening of one of his new libraries in 1905, and although there was a whiff of personal glory about his altruism, the funding provided by Carnegie and other philanthropists helped to establish public libraries outside of the industrial conurbations, areas in which provision was exclusively concentrated at the time.

The progressive, emancipatory spirit that had given rise to free book lending in the Victoria and Edwardian eras continued to drive the development of the public library in the post-war period. This was a time of consolidation and reconstruction during which the supply of books in circulation increased, as did the construction of new library buildings. With the advent of the landmark 1964 Public Libraries and Museums Act, which required every authority to provide 'comprehensive and efficient' library provision, the public library service had finally come into its own, with the decade between 1965 and 1975 being described as its 'golden age'. During this period central government invested heavily in the service, increasing expenditure in real terms by over 50 per cent, a boost in funding that dramatically transformed library provision: book stock and book loans soared and staff numbers increased by 40 per cent (colleges struggled to meet the surging demand for librarianship qualifications).

Yet even during this period of relative prosperity, the public service ethos of libraries continued to be challenged by reactionary voices who questioned the notion of information as a free public resource. There were calls for libraries to levy charges for their services, particularly the loan of fiction, the free availability of which was deemed to be an indulgent luxury unfairly subsidized by the taxpayer. Although core services continued to remain free of charge (book loans at least), government policies from the late 1970s were increasingly dedicated to a commercializing agenda which sought to introduce market mechanisms to the running of the public library. Pressures to commercialize came not only from central government but from a variety of policy units, foundations, watchdogs and research institutes that advocated the private ownership of information. In a consumer society, they argued, information was a commodity just like other goods and services, and the public library therefore should not be exempted from contributing to 'healthy' economic activity. All of which calls to mind the words of that ardent champion of the public library, Alan Bennett:

> On my walk I pass the Primrose Hill Community Library, which is closed to borrowers today but open for children, who throng the junior library, some of them sitting with an adult presumably learning to read, others in groups being told stories and at every table children reading on their own. This library is one of those institutions that Mark Littlewood, the head of the

right-wing think tank the Institute of Economic Affairs, said would make 'a useful retail outlet', a facility and a building for which there was no longer a social purpose. Most of the children reading here are black or Asian, with Somali children in the majority. As a so-called economist Littlewood presumably thinks the place would be better used as a Pizza Hut.

Bennett was writing at the beginning of 2015, by which time the public library had reached its present crisis point, a time when levels of funding were barely sufficient to maintain even a basic level of service. Not only had professional staff numbers plummeted such that libraries were now reliant on volunteers (between 2010 and 2015 the number of unpaid staff had risen by over 100 per cent, masking the concomitant reduction in qualified librarians), but also many libraries had been shut down and were continuing to close at an unrivalled rate. While some saw this as an unavoidable, if unfortunate, side effect of fiscal prudence, all part of the greater good of deficit reduction, others saw it for what it is: state-sanctioned social and cultural violence and the philistinization of local communities.

4

Against the current backdrop of cuts and closures, there have been calls for the public library to be overhauled if not dismantled altogether. In the eyes of some commentators, the rise of the internet and the ready availability of e-resources are rendering libraries obsolete, and hence we ought to question the state's obligation to maintain them. As the political strategist John McTernan puts it: 'Books are available for free from Project Gutenberg or for a small charge on Kindle. Second-hand books can be purchased from across the world via Alibris and Abebooks. As in so many other areas of life, as we get more prosperous we lean on public services less.'

Issues of cost and access aside, the digital imperative argument fails to recognize that a library is far more, of course, than a virtual collection of texts. Critics like McTernan overlook the fact that the public library is a unique space whose physical, social and cultural attributes cannot be replicated virtually. I doubt, too, that those who wish to radically overhaul the public library system appreciate the contribution that it makes to public health. Public libraries – and I suspect this is something librarians have known all along – are 'therapeutic landscapes', places conducive to recovery and the promotion of physical and psychological well-being.

Over the last twenty years or so, a growing body of research has demonstrated the positive impact that libraries have on people's health. One of the leading researchers in the field is Dr. Liz Brewster, a former librarian-turned-lecturer in medical education, who has been investigating the therapeutic potential of libraries for just under twenty years. Not long after my trip to Angel Row, I spoke to Brewster about her research. What was it about the public library, I wanted to know, that makes it conducive to restoration?

Libraries, she told me, are 'non-commercial, civic spaces that are open to anyone. You don't have to have any reason to be there. You don't have to have any excuse. And that fundamental ability simply to go in and browse the shelves is definitely undervalued. But it's not just about the books – it's the environment.'

In her research, Brewster has shown how the library was often a lifeline for people recovering from mental health problems. For these individuals, the library served as a haven, a calming space to which they could readily return during episodes of acute emotional distress. No matter how they interacted with the environment, the library was a place in which they were able to engage in ongoing acts of self-care. As Brewster put it:

It was that freedom of choice that the library afforded, something they could actively choose to do, something that was non-threatening if they were feeling particularly low. If they could go to the library, they wouldn't necessarily be challenged or forced to do something or made to buy something if they didn't have any money – they could just go, have a look, maybe choose some books, maybe not, maybe just have a sit and enjoy the atmosphere.

According to the wider 'spaces of care' literature – and Brewster's research is no exception – one of the hallmarks of therapeutic landscapes is their non-institutional nature. Although institutions in name, libraries are not seen as controlling, regulating spaces but as places free from the stigma associated with other public sanctuaries, such as shelters and hostels. For the socially excluded and dispossessed, the library is a place where they can settle into some form of civic life. In a study that examined homeless men's use of the public library, Darrin Hodgetts and colleagues describe how a visit to the library was, for the men concerned, a stabilizing event, a vital element of their daily routine which not only afforded them respite from homelessness but, as one of the participants put it, gave them the opportunity simply 'to read books and do what everyone else uses the library for, to read and have time out'.

Unqualified access to a space of care offers a resource for personal meaning and identity. In Hodgetts's study the homeless men were able to shed their maligned status as 'streeties' at the entrance to the library and, once inside, assume the mantle of 'ordinary' patron, experiencing a sense of belonging denied to them in other public places. Similarly, Brewster's participants were drawn to the library because of its inclusive atmosphere, an environment that afforded them a measure of social contact absent in other social settings. They described the positive relationships they'd developed with library staff (who knew them by name) and how they'd felt comfortable enough to make the staff aware of their problems. Even when they were experiencing such acute periods of turmoil that, to quote of the participants, the 'last thing on earth' they wanted to do was to 'have a chat with somebody', they nevertheless still craved company (albeit at a distance), still wished to be present among people and 'to see the same faces'.

5

It hardly needs to be said that the foregoing accounts are at odds with the popular conception of the public library as a silent and sombre place, a kind of secular cathedral inhabited by the lone scholar. Nowadays libraries are just as much about social capital as they are about silence and reflection. As Bella Bathurst argues, the 'great unsold truth' of modern public libraries is that people use them 'not because they're all about study, but because they're about connection. Connection with other worlds and points of view, even if that's no more than being among other people thinking and breathing.'

Even serious scholars aren't immune to the lure of bustly communal fellowship. Writing about the experience of researching his first book in the reading room ('315') of the New York Public Library, the literary critic Alfred Kazin described how he valued reading and working out his ideas 'in the midst of that endless crowd walking out of 315 looking for *something*', where the presence of the crowd was both an inspiring fillip and a consoling source of inclusion. In the equalizing context of the public library, there among the 'street philosophers, advertising salesman and the homeless', he was, he felt, 'one of the people', similarly seeking opportunity or merely getting on with life.

(Like Kazin, I'm impelled by civic bustle, cannot, in fact, work productively in the library without it, find absolute silence too oppressive, too exacting – it raises the stakes on industry, demands too much of me.)

Although some of Brewster's participants regretted the fact that the public library was no longer a quiet place, they nonetheless spoke of the appeal of a populated environment, a space in which they were aware that lives besides their own were being acted out and that, if even at a distance, they were in some way connected to them. Knowing that other patrons were doing the same kind of things as they were transformed the solitary activities of reading and reflection into a form of civic enterprise, an act of tacit communion. Only in the public library was it possible, it seemed, to reconcile the need for social contact with the need for solitude and seclusion.

When I asked Brewster what effect the recent library closures would have on communities, she was adamant that they'd be detrimental to public health: 'People *will* suffer,' she said. And what would aggravate the problem, she continued, was that those displaced users who depend on the library would struggle to avail themselves of alternative services of support. For when a library closes, what users report missing most of all is the physical space of the library, the atmosphere and environment of the place – the library as a social meeting point – features and attributes that uniquely contribute to enhancing well-being and quality of life. To close any library is to create 'a physical and social gap in the community'. ('I don't know of anything more disheartening than the sight of a shut down library,' lamented the poet and U. S. Laureate Charles Simic.) Whichever way you see it, closing libraries and reducing opening hours is a false economy. Retrenchment will certainly help councils make quick and easy savings, but will just as surely cause huge and irreparable damage to communities in the long term.

6

Towards the end of my visit to Angel Row, I sat at my old desk for a while. After reacquainting myself with the view out the window – steel staircases, vertical access ladders (not too much to waylay the eye) – I found myself reaching for the shelves, as I used to do. One of the books I pulled down was *The Pleasure of Reading*, a delightful collection of essays by famous authors describing their reading and literary influences. In one stand-out piece by

Doris Lessing (favourite books: Homer's *Iliad*, Gogol's *The Overcoat*, Woolf's *To the Lighthouse*), Lessing argued that public libraries are the most democratic things in the world ('What can be found there has undone dictators and tyrants') and wondered whether their neglect was because 'people who have access to good libraries, to history, ideas, information, cannot be told what to think. People who love literature have at least a part of their minds immune from indoctrination.'

I doubt I would have appreciated Lessing's argument when I first started using the library all those years ago. But it struck me now that all the time I'd spent at Angel Row was just as much a reaction against the conditioning effect of certain elements of police culture (insularity, machismo, conservatism) as it was evidence of a late intellectual awakening. A number of my police colleagues viewed reading – serious reading – with suspicion. To evince a love for bookish things was dangerous: you ran the risk of exposing yourself as an outsider, a crank who didn't fit in, at least with the alpha crowd, and it was the alpha crowd – the bully boys and their canteen culture – that troubled me the most. (If I ever left a book lying about, a book of poetry especially, chances were I would find it defaced on my return: oaths scrawled across the cover, pages ripped out.) Yet although being bookish risked derision, my appetite for reading continued unabated. I was learning to think for myself, to question the status quo. Reading granted me access to 'an alternative world, a way of living apart', in an often harsh and stultifying environment. Secretly making my way through *The Penguin Essays of George Orwell* and Larkin's *Collected Poems* was so much more interesting than taking part in office banter and the 'toad work' of processing petty criminals.

What would have happened to me if I hadn't found the library? I can't really answer that question. What I can say, however, is that the more I tramped the city streets all those years ago, the more I realized how empty and unfulfilled I was. I suppose I'd been obtuse and detached – too slow to appreciate that I wasn't cut out for police work, that I'd been adrift for years. It would be an exaggeration to claim that the library saved my life, but in providing ready access to a space of sanctuary and opportunity, a space where I was free of the myriad distractions and aggravations awaiting me outside, it lit up an escape route. I had no idea where this path would lead. I was just glad it was there.

3

Reawakening the mind: Poetry and the new culture of dementia care

If we are looking for areas in which people with dementia might excel,
then we may have found one in the arts.

– JOHN KILLICK

Poetry in the dark

One December evening, in 2013, the essayist and novelist Alberto Manguel sat down at his desk to write a letter. Just as he was about to put pen to paper, he felt as if his words were escaping him – rebelling, as he puts it – vanishing before he was able to get them down on the page. He was surprised but not too concerned, putting his word-finding difficulties down to fatigue, and promising himself he would rest as soon as he had finished the letter. But no matter how hard he tried to summon them, the words continued to elude him. When he went to tell his partner that something was wrong, he found that his speech was similarly compromised ('I was unable to mouth the words, except in a painfully protracted stutter'). A short while later he was in casualty, being treated for a stroke.

In order to satisfy himself that he hadn't lost his ability to recall words, only that of producing them, Manguel, as he lay in a darkened hospital room, began to reel off in his head stretches of literature that he knew by heart. What came forth most fluently, almost effortlessly, was poetry – great stretches of it – and in no time at all his mind was filled with the reassuring rhythms and rhymes of Edgar Allan Poe, Dante, and Victor Hugo.

Not long after this self-recital Manguel began to recover his linguistic abilities: within a few hours he was able to write again, and then, over the course of the following four or five weeks, his speech returned, free of all impediments bar a very slight stammer.

I've read Manguel's account of his stroke many times. What always affects me most about it – and this is not to take pleasure in his misfortune in any way – is the image of the stricken bibliophile lying in the darkness of his hospital room, in such terrifyingly uncertain circumstances, calling up and seeking succour in poetry, his faithful companion in the gloom. I like to think that as well as assuring him of his ability to remember words, Manguel's self-recital was a catalyst to his recovery – the internalized metrics of Poe and Hugo relieving him of the effects of what might otherwise have been a more severe and enduring dementia.

Of course, this is fanciful thinking. The (less romantic) reality is that Manguel's recovery would have involved the interplay of various factors – biological, pharmacological, social, cultural – associated with healing. Yet, as the poet and doctor Rafael Campo argues, 'there is something undeniably important about the role of words' in the recovery process, and Manguel's story hints at the therapeutic potential of literary discourse, poetry in particular. There is something peculiar to poetry that lends itself to aspects of healing and recovery, a quality that is perhaps most powerfully evinced in the context of dementia care.

As with other arts therapies that respond not just to the disease but the whole person, the therapeutic role of poetry in dementia is premised on the assumption that creative expression enhances cognitive function, capitalizing on the social and emotional abilities of people with the syndrome. Poetry therapy is able to conjure thoughts, emotions and memories – to bring the very 'surviving "self" to the fore' – such that the disease, if only momentarily, can be seen to give way to the person. This is something I have witnessed myself on countless occasions, and to experience it first-hand is always to be reminded that, even if the outer signs seem to betray an inner lifelessness, an apparent absence of soul and personality, there is always a deeper being beneath the disease.

The new culture of dementia care

Dementia is commonly understood in terms of loss: loss of memory, loss of language, loss of reason, and ultimately, supposedly, loss of self (a litany of depletion that is often reflected in the stark titles of popular books on the subject: *The Longest Loss, The Loss of Self, The Theft of Memory*, to name a few). In clinical terms, dementia is defined as a chronic neurodegenerative syndrome which arises as a result of some underlying disease of the brain, leading to the progressive loss of memory, language, thinking and orientation. Although the cause of dementia is not fully known (it cannot be simply reduced to genetics, age and lifestyle), the condition always involves some element of physical or chemical alteration of the brain, resulting in a reduction of neurons and brain volume.

Contrary to common belief, dementia is not a single disease per se but a syndrome, a collection of associated symptoms attributed to one or more underlying causes. Thus there are many specific forms of dementia, such as frontotemporal dementia, vascular dementia, and dementia with Lewy bodies, although the most common type is Alzheimer's disease, which accounts for approximately 75 per cent of all cases. To date, pharmaceutical remedies have had little impact on treating dementia. While some people appear to respond to treatment (e.g. looking more alert or seeming more focused), for others there will be no beneficial effect. Regardless of whether people's symptoms improve or not, there is no evidence that any drug currently in use is able to check the progression of dementia.

In the absence of any cure or effective clinical treatment, to be diagnosed with dementia is to be subject to what many believe to be a virtual death sentence – consigned to a life of passivity and withdrawal in the face of relentless deterioration. So common is this perception that the dementia rights activist Kate Swaffer has coined a term for it, 'Prescribed Disengagement®', a wry appellation which, as the patent symbol announces, she has successfully registered as a trademark, an officially branded way of being. 'Dementia is the only disease or condition I know of,' she argues, 'where patients are told to go home and give up their pre-diagnosis lives, rather than "to fight for their lives".'

Writing from personal experience (she is currently living with early-onset dementia, having been diagnosed at the age of forty-nine), Swaffer describes how, on receiving her diagnosis, she was advised by her healthcare providers to give up work and focus instead on putting in place end-of-life plans, advice which, if she'd heeded, would have sanctioned a life of fear and hopelessness. 'Having dementia does not mean you have to give up living a pre-diagnosis life,' she writes. 'Dementia may well be a terminal illness and feel like a death sentence when we are first diagnosed, but we don't have to die straight away.'

Of course, not all health care providers prescribe disengagement, and those who do no doubt believe they are acting in their patients' best interests. But the treatment and understanding of dementia continue to be dominated by a medical model that reaches for clinical rather than human-centred responses. Broadly speaking, the medical model treats dementia as a biological phenomenon, an organic brain disorder, and accordingly tends to focus on the pathology itself rather than the individual affected by the syndrome, as though dementia and its effects on a person's health and behaviour were attributable to brain composition alone.

Yet, as the late, great Tom Kitwood argued, such an approach leaves social and interpersonal factors out of the picture. Kitwood, a psychologist who revolutionized the field of dementia care, was one of the first researchers to argue that the social environment can significantly affect the well-being of people with dementia. A poor care environment, he claimed, can accelerate the dementing process, while a flourishing one can bring about 'rementing', the partial recovery of certain powers assumed to be irrevocably lost.

Kitwood believed that people with dementia always retain their essential humanity. He was one of the first researchers to challenge the commonly held view that having the disease entails the loss of self, the complete erosion of personality and identity. Not all the symptoms of the syndrome, he argued, are due to pathological changes in the brain. Some are due to what he called 'malignant social psychology', a set of often unconscious attitudes and actions that demean and dehumanize people with dementia, such as treating them as objects or preventing them from harnessing their remaining powers, attitudes and actions liable to undermine the standing of the individual and precipitate further cognitive decline. It was therefore vital to treat dementia not as a disease but as a disability, the severity of which is determined by the quality of care people receive.

When Kitwood first aired his theories in the late 1980s, it was near sacrilege to claim that dementia was anything but a manifestation of brain disease. As Professor Bob Woods, a fellow psychologist and contemporary of Kitwood, puts it, 'Tom always had to battle with the establishment in order for his ideas to be accepted', and even now it feels mildly subversive, in the face of biomedical orthodoxy, to restate and advance his arguments. Nevertheless, despite initial objections and subsequent critical reappraisals, Kitwood's theories have become more widely accepted. Today a new culture of care has emerged, a more person-centred approach that no longer regards people with dementia in isolation from their social environment. The legacy of Kitwood's work has been to show how, with the right kind of support, it is possible to maintain one's sense of self and self-esteem in the face of cognitive decline – a legacy which, twenty years after his death, now forms the basis of best practice in contemporary dementia care.

In search of a reading group

The advent of the new culture of care has given rise to a flourishing of activities aimed at improving the lives of people with dementia. Much has been written about the value of arts interventions in the dementia research literature – music and reminiscence therapies in particular. Much less is known about the therapeutic role that poetry can play in dementia care. This is surprising, given that many of the benefits attributed to music and other therapies can be brought about by poetry. As with music, for example, the response to poetry appears to be preserved in people with dementia: if, as Oliver Sacks has shown in his celebrated *Musicophilia*, we retain a memory, a sensibility for rhythm and melody, then it's not unreasonable to assume that we also possess a poetic memory, one stimulated by lexical and phonetic patterning, the irresistible alchemy of words and language.

This predisposition for poetry is something that the former poet laureate Andrew Motion, a long-standing advocate of poetry therapy, has often written about. 'I'm not a neuroscientist,' he told me during an email correspondence, 'but it seems as though the brains of our species are hard-wired to retain and enjoy the characteristic features of poetry. We might happen to grow up to enjoy speaking about poetry in a complex and sophisticated way – and to writing it similarly. But truly the appeal it makes to us is basic and fundamental. We are a poetic species. Poetry is like breathing to us.'

Indeed, for Motion, it was the characteristic features of poetry that first got him pondering the relationship between dementia and the therapeutic potential of words. As he put it:

> When my mother was ill and in hospital through my late teens and twenties I noticed (although she didn't have dementia) how much pleasure (though not a 'literary' person) she took in reading and hearing poems. Rhyme and strong rhythm seemed to make a very primitive appeal to her, and whenever she remembered poems from her childhood it seemed she was encountering treasure that she especially valued.
>
> This laid the foundation of my interest in thinking about how poetry helps ill people. Then a few years ago I was approached to become the president of an organization called Kissing It Better … which sends secondary school children into care homes to sing and recite poems to people with dementia. I gladly accepted the role and went on a few visits with the kids – and was always astonished by the effect of these little performances. Again, the primitive appeal of rhythm and rhyme was able to cut through or across all sorts of impediments to full consciousness, and to release and revive other poems that the patients had lurking in their memories. Really very seriously upset people would become (though generally briefly) lucid and happy.

That cutting-through-to-consciousness is one of the essences of poetry therapy. Indeed, it was the phenomenon that, more than anything else, I had hoped to reproduce when I first started reading in dementia care settings. I thought, as Motion's account intimates, that it would simply be a matter of reciting poems and then stepping back to appreciate the intended effects – the participants animated, engaged, brought back to themselves. I thought that reading aloud communally would, moreover, connect people who, despite having lived under the same roof for years, might never have conversed or spent much meaningful time together. But my first attempts at poetry therapy were disappointing.

Inspired by accounts like Motion's, I'd long wanted to set up a dementia reading group. In order to do so, I'd approached one of the many care homes near to where I live and, such was the enthusiasm of the management, quickly established a weekly run group there. The home – let us call it 'Larch Meadow' – was a privately owned establishment, tucked away, to adopt the brochure-speak, in a quiet and secluded suburban area. The management seemed progressive in outlook and were keen to include new pursuits in their daily round of activities. The atmosphere of the place seemed calm and dignified, courtly even, an ambience partly owing to the presence of a large reminiscence space in which a variety of vintage objects – telephone and wireless circa 1940, spinning top, Pears Transparent Soap, Silver Jubilee regalia – were reverently laid out in elegant museum-like display cases. The staff to-and-froing through the public lobby, and twinkling on cue, appeared unfazed and purposeful. Through certain windows and a wide set of French doors one glimpsed a well-tended garden, which, according to the shiny prospectus, the residents enjoyed helping to maintain.

It quickly became apparent, however, that the day-to-day operations of the place were not as impeccable as the front stage facade suggested. In fact the conditions there, in some respects, were more like those witheringly described in the classic sociological critiques of residential care settings in the 1950s and 1960s than the person-centred conditions that one would expect as a matter of course in the twenty-first century. The home had a high turnover of care workers and was clearly understaffed. The manager was rarely on the premises, preferring, it seemed, to 'work' from home (like Shakespeare's Rosaline, she was spoken about but never actually seen). The only ever-present member of staff was the apologetically harried activities coordinator who – understandably in the face of the depleted workforce – was keen to offload as many residents onto me as possible. This meant that I often worked with large numbers of participants, several of whom resented being pitchforked into the poetry sessions – 'It's like being back at school, isn't it?' – grouching and harrumphing throughout.

Matters were aggravated by our never having access to a quiet space. The room I'd originally been promised – which, in every regard, was perfect for reading aloud: quiet, comfortable, intimate – was never made available to me. Instead, I had to use the TV lounge, which at that time in the morning was already half full of residents, most of whom spent their entire day there. They sat about dozing in wing-back chairs or, if awake, tamely enduring the vacuous assault of daytime television, against which the inspiriting rhythms of Robert Browning and Edgar Allan Poe had little chance of working their magic … (For sworn believers in the affirming power of poetry, few things are more soul-destroying than having to recite 'How They Brought the Good News from Ghent to Aix' over the ambient din of *Homes Under the Hammer*.)

I gave up going to Larch Meadow after about three to four weeks.

By heart

There is a moment – in fact, it is *the* moment – in Gillian Clarke's poem 'Miracle on St David's Day' when a psychiatric patient, long rendered mute by severe depression, suddenly begins to speak again. (The events narrated are based on a true story, a reading that Clarke gave at a South Wales hospital in the 1970s.)

> He is suddenly standing, silently,
> huge and mild, but I feel afraid. Like slow
> movement of spring water or the first bird
> of the year in the breaking darkness,
> the labourer's voice recites 'The Daffodils'.

The nurses are frozen, alert; the patients
seem to listen. He is hoarse but word-perfect.
Outside the daffodils are still as wax,
a thousand, ten thousand, their syllables
unspoken, their creams and yellows still.

Forty years ago, in a Valleys school,
the class recited poetry by rote.
Since the dumbness of misery fell
he has remembered there was a music
of speech and that once he had something to say.

In the care homes I subsequently read at, where conditions were far more conducive to reading aloud, I regularly witnessed similar reawakenings and began to appreciate the powerful effect poetry can have on memory, mood, and cognition. It was extremely moving to see otherwise agitated or inert individuals calmed or quickened, to see them warming to poems first encountered generations ago but still preserved in the mind's clear amber and recalled with great facility and precision.

The effect was always the same. As soon as I read the opening lines of a familiar poem aloud, there was a collective stirring, a shift in orientation: heads lifted or turned towards me and then, after a moment tuning into the recital and picking up the thread, the listeners would begin to recite the poem for themselves – tentatively and discretely at first, but then with increasing vigour and confidence until they were all in step with each other, a perfectly synchronized chorus.

When they were in full flight like this, firmly etched into a groove, I would stop reading, withdrawing, as it were, my undertow of support, allowing them to free wheel and complete the recital in their own time and after their own fashion. On such occasions not only were they able to recite poems in their entirety, they were also able to recover various moods and memories intimately associated with them, often in acute sensory detail. A poem such as John Masefield's 'Sea Fever', for example, with its suggestive refrain ('I must go down to the seas again …') would invariably open the floodgates to a stream of vivid recollections of seaside holidays and excursions, the lines acting, in Oliver Sacks's phrase, as a kind of 'Proustian mnemonic', as well as seemingly heightening the participants' linguistic and sensory facilities – as their various long-forgotten but vividly recalled impressions often made evident: the experience of walking barefoot along a beach ('the feel of shingle beneath my feet'), the ambience of shabby guest houses ('the dusty smell of the place').

These reminiscences, moreover, no matter how disparate, were likely to prompt further recollections: one memory would trigger another, then another, each complementing and extending its predecessor – memories both squarely staying on, and jubilantly straying off, topic. In this chain-like fashion, groups would light on subjects as broad and particular as where they grew up, the schools they went to and the places where they worked. Nights at the Palais de Danse and visits to stern aunts. Larders and pantries. Sunday dinner in the front room (used once a week, and for that purpose only). Making a fire on cold winter mornings. Walking in bluebell woods …

During the exchange of all these memories and impressions, I recalled comments by the gerontologist Henk Loning, a specialist in nursing home care. Writing apropos of group reminiscence therapy, specifically with regard to the use of old photographs to stimulate recollection, Loning observes how older people living in residential care are compelled to enter into dependent relationships, but during conversations about historical photographs that dependency ebbs away – to the point where they become experts on the images – experts in the sense that, provided with a powerful visual connection to the past, they are uniquely able to inform others about personal memories that the old pictures bring to the surface.

In a not dissimilar vein, my participants, as they teased out personal meanings and associations in familiar poems, achieved a kind of private expertise, revealing in the process a heightened sense of self-confidence rarely occasioned by other facets of the care home regimen. This was particularly the case, perhaps not surprisingly, with participants who had a lifelong love of poetry, but who had lost their appetite for reading or were no longer able to read.

One such resident was Eileen. When I first met Eileen, she had only recently been admitted to residential care and, as is often the case when people relocate to assisted living, was struggling to adapt to her new environment. The adjustment was proving particularly difficult for Eileen, since she had spent virtually all her life in the family home, continuing to live there after her parents had died. She was happy in the family house, which she adored and where she maintained an intimate connection with the past, not least her beloved parents, whom she missed intensely. 'I shall be going home, shan't I?' she would ask over and over, soliciting anyone and everyone within earshot. 'Do tell me I'm going home, won't you please? I miss it so much.'

What compounded Eileen's adjustment difficulties was that she had neither friends nor family (at any rate she never received any visitors, and no one called after her). Except for a few possessions transferred to her new room, where she spent most of her day, emerging only for meals and the occasional activity, Eileen had lost virtually all association with her former life and the world outside. She had no one to assist or advocate for her, no one to help ease her into and support her through this difficult period of adjustment. (It is well known that the involvement of family and friends can mitigate the trauma of transition – particularly for residents who are unable to express their needs or might otherwise be excluded from decision-making.)

The residents didn't take to Eileen at first. They were wary of her, put out by her ceaseless importuning and unsettling agitation, and were quick to disabuse her of any notion of her returning home. They told her she would never be going back, that she lived here now, whereupon, as if receiving the news for the first time, she would burst into tears, only a moment later to resume her importuning again – and then again to receive the same response. (On and on it went, a never-ending loop of hope and heartbreak.)

I was uncertain how to answer to Eileen's entreaties. I admired the practised way the staff mollified her, the way they distracted her from the gnawing itch of her idée fixe, either by subtly shifting the emphasis of conversation (without changing the subject completely) or by drawing her attention to some diverting aspect of the home environment. As an outsider, and someone who hardly knew Eileen at the time, I felt unable to deploy either strategy. And so, in order to avoid breaking her heart whenever she fired her eternal question at me, I did the only thing I could do. I read a poem.

How to describe the change that came over Eileen? Sometimes it was instant, corresponding with the point at which I started reading; at other times it was gradual, halting, with her taking a little time first to apprehend the switch in spoken register – the sudden shift from conversational to literary discourse – before giving herself over to the recital completely. She was calm, receptive, her face pressed into an expression of motionless concentration, as if to shut out everything except for the words of the poems which, whether she appeared to know them or not, held her as though in a trance – a reverie which would persist for as long as I continued to read aloud to her. 'Was that Walter de la Mare?' she asked. '"The Listeners"? Do you have any Hilaire Belloc – "The South Country"? Oh, I do love poetry!' Eileen, it soon transpired, had an extensive poetic repertoire, knew long stretches of verse by heart and would take great delight in reciting her favourite poets at length, her otherwise brittle-anxious voice ringing out, to much applause, in the little activities room where we were all gathered.

Yet it would be an exaggeration to claim that, although transfiguring while it lasted, the effect of the poetry on Eileen was long lived. For once the poems had stopped, she would withdraw into herself, become quiet and glassy-eyed and ask to be taken back to her room. (I wondered, somewhat fancifully, whether it might be possible to engineer a poetic drip-feed for her, some means of connecting her to poetry for hours at a time, so as to maintain her transformation for longer. But I never came up with anything.)

Sometimes when I turned up with my rattle bag of poems, Eileen was reluctant to leave her room. On such occasions, rather than join the other residents in the activities suite, the two of us would relocate to a quiet area on the first floor landing ('a pair of outcasts', she called us), and again I would be struck by the change that came over her and the quickening influence of the poetry, both of us losing all sense of time and space during these brief encounters, such that when one of the staff came to announce that it was midday, time for Eileen to go down to lunch, it was as though we were being summoned from somewhere else, another place altogether, a place to which we never wished to return.

Poetry on the brain

Julie Walker, a UK-based bibliotherapist, emailed me recently about an experience she'd had in one of her workshops:

> It can often be very difficult to know whether people are engaging with poetry. I look for the more subtle and less obvious indications that someone is engaged … One lady in a care home was a regular at my sessions, though I felt that the staff brought her to me rather than her coming of her own volition. She was very withdrawn, rarely made eye contact with anyone and had lost the power of speech. At one session I read 'Night Mail' by W. H. Auden ['This is the Night Mail crossing the Border, / Bringing the cheque and the postal order …'] and noticed that she was rocking in time to the rhythm of the poem. I chose more poems with a distinct rhythm and she

either rocked or tapped her hand on the arm of the chair in perfect time to the poems.

Rhythm, neurologists inform us, harnesses the 'very foundational, subcortical levels of the brain'. It is not surprising, therefore, that certain forms of motor memory and motor response (as evidenced in coordinated movement such as dancing, foot-tapping, and so on) invariably survive to some degree in even the severest of dementias. The response to rhythm, moreover, is never purely mechanical. The coordinated, perfectly timed rocking and tapping that Julie describes is surely testament to a sensible, appreciative reaction to rhythm, a felt response to what Samuel Taylor Coleridge called the 'intoxicating' influence of metre. For Coleridge, metre was the chief instrument and source of visceral stimulation in poetry (pleasure in and of itself, according to the great Romantic, being the principal object of verse) with poetic metre acting as a mental and physical stimulant, increasing 'the vivacity and susceptibility of the general feelings and of the attention'.

But as well as a sharpened sensibility, Julie's account also evinces the heightened social connectivity that metrical stimulation can bring about: to embody and to be attuned to metre is not only to (re)activate certain perceptual and cognitive capacities but also, in this communal context, to be in contact with and to align oneself with others. As Julie herself concluded:

> My participant raised her head and briefly looked at me at the end of the session. I felt that the poems had helped her to reconnect with the world and the people around her; to share in an experience, to be a participant rather than a mere presence.

***

Although it plays an important role, metre is only one formal element that stimulates and helps people connect with poetry. With its recurring accents and patterns, its sounds arranged in and through time, metre shares certain properties with music. But though musical in various respects, metered poetry (indeed all poetry), as David Constantine reminds us, is never music. The sounds and rhythms of poetry also convey meaning, 'are charged with precise lexical sense and, most often, come trailing centuries of connotations'. Poetry is a distinctive blend of sound and sense, and some neuroscientists and literary critics have argued that it is this interplay between the acoustic and semantic that accounts for poetry's powerful psychological and physiological effects.

To be sure, poetry, as with any sensory input, does things to the brain. As Frederick Turner and Ernst Pöppel write in their classic paper 'The Neural Lyre: Poetic Meter, the Brain and Time':

> The musical and pictorial powers of the right brain are enlisted by meter to cooperate with the linguistic powers of the left; and by auditory driving effects, the lower levels of the nervous system are stimulated in such a way as to reinforce the cognitive functions of the poem, to improve the memory, and to promote physiological and social harmony.

In other words, poetry introduces the creative processes associated with the right hemisphere of the brain into its logical, language-processing counterpart, the left hemisphere. Or to put it another way, 'poetry gives both sides of our brain an "equal opportunity"'. But Turner and Pöppel go further, arguing that not only does poetry have the capacity to tickle both hemispheres, but that it is also fundamentally aligned with human psychology. They argue that lines of metered poetry, in all languages and cultures, tend to be of a fixed duration, a predictable span of between 2.5 and 3.5 seconds when spoken aloud. On the basis of this three-second postulate, they suggest that the underpinning master-rhythm of all human poetry is not pulmonary but neural, with poets and readers subconsciously composing and processing poetry in three-second 'parcels of experience'. So assured are Turner and Pöppel of the brain's alignment with the duration of verse lines that they describe poetic meter as the pre-eminent cognitive enhancer, a kind of cerebral ambrosia that, among other things, stimulates 'the brain's capacities for self-reward' and 'nicely fulfills' its habitual need for novelty.

Fascinating and pluckily ingenious though their theory is, it is one thing to measure the average duration of various lines of poetry; quite another to claim that our neural system is in perfect accord with the length of a line of verse. For a start, it is of course debatable whether all lines of poetry universally elapse within a three-second window. The authors don't properly take into account the actual manner of articulation (the duration of any spoken verse line depends on the performer delivering it and to what end their delivery) and base their theory of temporal constraint on a relatively modest collection of poems. Moreover, for all their recourse to neuroscientific precepts, their study remains somewhat speculative – they offer little empirical evidence with which to verify their neuro-poetic claims, relying on conjecture and intuition.

Since the publication of Turner and Pöppel's famous 1983 paper, which is still often cited by scholars from various fields, an increasing number of studies have taken up the challenge to put poetry on a secure neural footing. Two elements characterize this body of research: first, it harnesses ever more sophisticated neuroimaging technologies to illuminate (literally) people's physiological and neural responses to poetry; and second, it is interdisciplinary in nature, bringing together researchers from both sides of the so-called 'two cultures' divide. An illustrative example is Noreen O'Sullivan and colleagues' (2015) study which uses fMRI (functional magnetic resonance imaging) to compare the differential effects that both poetry and prose have on the brain. The authors begin with the assumption that the processing of more verbally intricate texts is liable to bring about changes in cognition that can enhance well-being (engaging with more nuanced meanings in texts, they suggest, promotes the adoption of more fluid and adaptive ways of thinking). Peering into the crania of twenty-four poetry- and prose-reading participants, O'Sullivan et al. show how poetry activates more lateral frontal and temporal-occipital regions of the brain than prose is observed to do. This activation, they claim, is consistent with the idea that reading poetry requires appraising numerous threads of meaning and hence requires more focused attention, the flexing of a wider range of neural mechanisms.

Of particular significance is the recruiting of the caudate nucleus, a part of the brain that appears to play a pivotal role in the processing of poetic texts. As one of the paper's authors, Philip Davis, a professor of English literature, explained to me (I'd consulted Davis for a clearer understanding of his study, the finer details of which, for a non-neurologist, are not always easy to appreciate): 'The left caudate nucleus does the work of recognising at its top part. At its bottom part, it is a reward mechanism. What is great about it is that it isn't like a mechanism because it does the two things [recognising and rewarding] – simultaneously. So if you recognise a surprise in poetry, the actual act makes you feel good.'

It is this propensity for neural reward – the payoff for processing dynamic meaning – that is compromised in people experiencing cognitive impairment. 'Therefore the hypothesis in our paper,' Davis continued, 'is that if people get more used to reading literature that has those surprises that require something other than the mechanical, the more they can do that, the more those parts of the brain that are under-activated, undernourished, begin to work and begin to give them pleasure.'

I like this hypothesis. But how seriously should we take this kind of neuroimaging research? One particularly knotty issue is that the difference between poetry and prose is by no means absolute. Certain strains of prose – so-called poetic prose or the prose poem – share many of the formal characteristics found in poetry (rhythm, assonance, consonance, metaphor, and so on), while some poems read more like segmented prose than conventional poetry. This formal uncertainty, moreover, is exacerbated by the fact that there has long been, and continues to be, disagreement about what poetry actually is. For centuries, countless scholars and practitioners have attempted to pinpoint the essence of poetic form: 'the best words in the best order' (Coleridge); 'nothing else than the most perfect speech of man' (Arnold); 'a composition of words set to music' (Ezra Pound); 'memorable speech' (Auden) – all of which, of course, might equally apply to certain strains of prose.

As these stabs at a definition suggest, poetry is a value-laden term, tied up with personal judgements that themselves are a reaction to shifting literary and historical trends. Not surprisingly, this conceptual uncertainty poses problems of interpretation for neuroimaging studies, which, for the sake of experimentation, tend to treat poetry as a discrete entity, a linguistic variety naturally distinct and distinguishable from other modes of writing.

This is a point that the philosopher Raymond Tallis, long-standing scourge of what he calls 'neuromania' – namely, the idea 'that the best way of understanding human beings is to examine their brain activity' – has repeatedly made. For Tallis, neuroimaging reveals very little about the experience of poetry – any more than it reveals anything interesting about highly subjective concepts such as love, hatred, or wisdom. 'It's not useful to try to map on to a bodily organ that has evolved distinctions that are highly cultural,' he tells me. 'What counts as poetry and what counts as prose will be disputed forever.'

Tallis is not critical of neuroimaging per se, which yields important insights into the workings of the human brain. Rather, he is dismissive of claims that the impact of human culture can be explained simply by probing neural pathways – that brain mechanics alone can account for the various effects that literature, painting, music, and other arts have on people.

'There is of course some kind of correlation between brain activity and certain kinds of experience,' he observes, 'but it is so broad it would encompass things that aren't poetry or music – and therefore it doesn't really tell you anything about what is specific to the experience of poetry or music, even less what is specific to the experience of a particular poem by a particular person at a particular time.'

***

If, as Tallis argues, functional neuroimaging research contributes relatively little to our understanding and experience of poetry, it at least helps confirm, in revealing the extent and intensity of brain activation, what we already know about poetry: that it moves and excites us, that it transports and delights, that it beguiles, arouses, provokes, calms, confounds ... And in fairness to many neuroscientific studies (Turner and Pöppel being a notable exception), they do not presume to account for poetry in neurobiological terms entirely, and are, in truth, rather modest about their contribution to our understanding of literary texts, often highlighting various methodological limitations while calling for greater interdisciplinary collaboration in order to explain their findings and insights.

Indeed, even Professor Philip Davis, who has long worked at the interface of literary studies and neuroscience, is quick to acknowledge the shortcomings of brain scanning techniques when applied to literature. If brain imaging for him is as 'close to a representation of raw immediate experience as we're ever going to get', it is also, he observes, 'just one dimension among many – merely part of a gathering body of evidence' that helps to illuminate our responses to poetry and literature more widely.

For Davis, poetry, with its 'rhythms, jolts, and surprises', is the linguistic antidote par excellence to 'mental rigidification'. Poetry is a means of 'thinking about' and 'getting hold of existence' instead of 'being stuck in it'. When I ask him specifically how this relates to dementia, he tells me about an experiment run by the facilitator of a poetry group for older people. The facilitator, believing that continued exposure to a text enhances rather than diminishes its potency, wanted to see how participants responded to the repeated reading of a much-loved poem.

It was Wordsworth's daffodils, of course. I say 'of course' because it's often used, though the great thing about literature is if it's good, it bears repetition and doesn't feel repeated because it comes back again, and that's very, very important, as it were, about the quality of the thing.

Anyway, the experiment was this. She would read it to them again. Some people already knew the poem. Some people didn't. Some people remembered they'd done it a previous week. Some people didn't, as far as one could tell. What's interesting is that none of those differences made any difference in this sense. That people would either point from one session to another to different parts of the poem or in pointing to the same part of the poem would say somewhat different things about it.

This is important because in dementia you just get stuck in a particular formulation – sometimes in a particular memory – but vocabulary and point of view were changing.

This is extraordinary because it means that even in a poem that is already at some level known, it's still new, and that people here are responding to something new. So that instead of reminiscence therapy, which takes people back to material objects like, say, a ration book, which on the whole is designed to make people feel happy, this trigger in poetry takes people or brings their memory forward spontaneously without knowing what object it is – in the way you know what a ration book is – in ways that are not simply prescribed to be in inverted commas 'positive'.

He's on to something. To read a poem aloud to others repeatedly – to the point where you can barely bring yourself to recite it again – is always for someone to apprehend some meaning or detail they had yet to appreciate, or to provoke some quickening response in participants hitherto silent and detached. In other words, every reading of a poem is a first reading, since, if it is of sufficient quality at least, it will be liable to change in the minds of readers and listeners – will be a different poem on each occasion.

As Davis argues, it is only through regular re-reading that poetry is able 'to do testimony to people's deeper experiences'. Anything short of this sustained engagement with texts is unlikely to stimulate the mental powers of people with dementia in quite the same way – 'to produce,' as he puts it, 'those sorts of awakenings that themselves awaken respect in others who are suddenly able to see that the person is still there'. This combined awakening is, he concludes, especially important for friends and families of people with dementia – for they can see for themselves that their loved ones can still 'regularly, repeatedly, if unpredictably, come back from the deeper part of autobiographical memory … And that's encouraging.'

Dementia and the creative mind

Not long after my conversation with Davis, I paid a visit to my local community centre. Each week it hosts a Memory Café. Conceived by the Dutch psychologist Bère Miesen, Memory Cafés (also known as Alzheimer's and Dementia Cafés in other parts of the world) are a relatively new feature of British civic life, though nowadays a Café can be found in most towns and villages across the UK. 'Café' suggests cosey sociability. But Memory Cafés are not casual gatherings. They are structured get-togethers that feature talks and activities, gatherings where people with dementia and their supporters can meet and participate as equals. In such a supportive environment, participants can share experiences and insights, breaking free from the stigma that can lead to people with memory loss withdrawing from social situations and activities that they once enjoyed.

Each memory café meeting revolves around a different theme. Today's was poetry and I'd been invited along to observe the session and read a few poems. But the focus this afternoon was not so much on reading poetry as on making it. On tables scattered around the hall were poetry kits – packs containing strips of cut up words, sticks of glue and pieces of card – with which to make found poems. The beauty of creating found poems – texts assembled out of words and phrases culled from existing sources – is that it's an accessible but no less imaginative mode of composition that gives voice to those who might have lost, or are beginning to lose, confidence in their cognitive powers. While composing poems from scratch might be beyond the capacity of people with advanced dementia, found poems, with a little assistance if required, are relatively easy to create. There is no need for the poem to make grammatical or logical sense, or to aspire to any level of literary competence. Delightfully, anything goes.

The hall fills up quickly, the tables soon occupied. They are couples mainly – husbands, wives, partners, but also parents with supporting sons or daughters. I go from table to table, watching them at work. Each group has their own way of composing. Some begin by first picking out an alluring lexeme and then wrapping associated words around it. Others experiment more with chance, weaving together long strings of randomly selected words. Whatever their mode of composition, I'm struck by how indistinguishable the group members are from one another. Watching them work together – the collaborative way in which they weigh up and choose words, chuckle over absurd juxtapositions ('leafy communitarian', 'rivers of solar sushi') – it's impossible to tell the carers apart from those they care for. Although we are assembled in a dedicated dementia setting, dementia itself is somewhere else.

At the end of the afternoon, Gillian, the event organizer, invites me up to the microphone to read the found poems. Many of them are ludically epigrammatic, bringing about much laughter, while others give rise to short silences – poems that, in their thick concentration of nouns and noun phrases, have something of an imagist feel to them. All of the poems – and I say this without any whiff of condescension – are arresting in their own way and carry their own rhetorical energy. All are warmly applauded.

***

Reading the poems aloud that afternoon, and noticing their use of elaborate imagery, I was reminded of the fact that, far from fatally compromising creative expression, dementia can 'release' it. As the syndrome takes hold, literal language often gives way to an increasing use of metaphor, simile and other vivid turns of phrase. It is said to 'bloom' with symbol and allusion, to be driven by a creative disinhibition that 'sweeps away' barriers to self-expression.

Among dementia specialists, this is a view that reaches its apotheosis in the work of John Killick, a professional poet who has perhaps done more than any other creative writer to affirm the expressive capacities of people living with dementia. For over twenty years, Killick, a retired English teacher, has worked as writer in residence in care homes and hospitals, where out of the words of residents and patients, he has fashioned lyric and narrative poetry, much of which has found its way into published anthologies and magazines.

Working on the belief that 'the natural language of those with dementia is poetry', Killick's approach to composition involves first getting to know his subjects and then, after establishing a mutual rapport, eliciting their stories and experiences:

> I make it clear … they can talk about anything that interests them. At a certain point, when intimacy and fluency have been achieved, I may ask permission to write down or tape-record their words. Occasionally a poem is achieved then and there. Usually it is a matter of taking away their words and working on them. There is one important exception however (and this is the first golden rule): I add nothing, only take away.

Many of the resultant poems are richly figurative, betraying a desire, perhaps, to express feelings no longer communicable in literal language. The effect of these tropes is to bring language closer to perceived experience, and hence to the apparent significance of lived events. In the following poem, for instance, the recurring notion of kidnap and confinement, and its tantalizing proximity with freedom and possibility, immerses us in the emotional reality of the speaker:

Are we all kidnapped?
I'm not at all sure

what kidnapping is, but
I know I'm very frightened.

I could go out there
and sit on that swing
and I would enjoy it.
I want my freedom.

But we none of us have our freedom.
I don't understand so much
that I'll just do without it,
chuck the whole lot in the air.

In a postscript to *You are Words*, an anthology of dementia poetry that features the lines above, Killick recounts how he asked a literary critic for his opinion of the poems. The (unnamed) critic was somewhat sniffy, though not for literary-aesthetic reasons: he felt the poems were, and I quote, 'not mad enough'! Killick was simultaneously outraged and encouraged: the critic had evidently expected nonsense, but here was recognition of the difficulty of making 'black-and-white judgements' about madness and dementia, a tacit acknowledgement of the persistence of meaning in those presumed to be incapable of producing rational discourse. (In Killick's poems, one sees dementia not as a state of mindlessness but as a state of mind. His work challenges the idea that the syndrome destroys personality, encouraging us to imagine and empathize with the lives of people living with it.)

Yet, for all its humanizing effect, the question remains as to whose poetry it actually is. For even though the poet preserves the original vocabulary, the speaker's words are pressed into dedicated service: corralled and compressed into lines and stanzas to enhance their poetic resonance. Understandably, not all of Killick's subjects approve of their words being used in this way, as Killick himself concedes: 'As can be imagined, reactions to the poems may vary. At one extreme there can be a rejection of the poem as worthless or a denial of its authorship. At the other comes the injunction to publish: "Anything you can tell people about how things are for me is important."'

All thing considered, most people seem to enjoy the collaboration, valuing the chance to share their interior worlds with others. The writer John Berger speaks of poems crossing battlefields and tending to the wounded. Poetry, he writes, provides an assurance that 'language has acknowledged, has given shelter to … experience which demanded, which cried out'. And it's this vivid act of witness and testimony that's at the heart of Killick's poems. Whatever one thinks about their mode of composition, the poems give voice to the voiceless, confirm for them that 'their words are being taken seriously' and confirm for us, not that confirmation should be needed, that 'it is worth communicating with people with dementia', that dementia is no bar to meaningful exchange.

Envoi

A few months ago, I spoke at a local dementia forum on 'The psychological benefits of poetry'. It was a talk I'd given countless times before, had off pat, and so on this occasion, a relatively informal affair, I was surprised to find myself suddenly very nervous, close, in fact, to the point of bolting. Rather than linger through my slides, freely expanding on points and developing an argument, I mumbled and quavered throughout, rarely looking up from my PowerPoint.

At the conference reception later in the afternoon, I was approached by a smartly dressed, stern-looking man.

'You shouldn't have given that talk,' he said.

Here we go again, I said to myself. (Throughout the day, I'd been accosted by various interlopers, each with their well-intentioned public speaking advice.)

'You shouldn't have given that talk,' he said again.

I told him I was sorry, that these things happen to the best of us.

'I looked after my wife for thirteen years,' he said, his voice faltering. 'I played music to her, sang with her, went dancing with her. But I never read poetry to her.'

Silence.

'She would've loved that.'

4

The enduring self: A journal

Tho' much is taken, much abides ...
– ALFRED LORD TENNYSON

In August 2015, I received an email from Susan and Rachel S. concerning their father, Robert, a retired lecturer in English literature. They had heard about my interest in poetry and dementia and wondered whether I would like to meet their dad, who, although 'he struggles to read and remember things', still 'loves literature and would probably enjoy talking about University and his time there'. I gladly accepted the invitation – the first of its kind I'd received – and began to visit Robert at his sheltered apartment, where I would spend increasing amounts of time reading and chatting to him. Although I wasn't to know it at the outset, our time together would develop into an enduring friendship, a friendship that would change the way I thought about dementia.

I learned many things from Robert – not least the fact that cognitive decline is by no means synonymous with the loss of the person – that the self persists – though the ways in which it reveals itself are often subtle and easy to overlook.

13 January 2016

My third meeting with Robert, who remains as genial and charming as ever. There is an aura, a warm and easy quiet about him – if that's the right way of putting it. At any rate, I no longer feel compelled to initiate small talk all the time, to stem the periodic flow of gaps and pauses. It's pleasant merely to sit with him, silently poring over poems and sipping tea: one doesn't necessarily need language to share an intimacy. Indeed, I often feel during these quiet moments that, to paraphrase Walter de la Mare, something more than words seems to pass between us, something beyond the reach of language.

This is not to say that he is without words. Although dementia has affected his speech – both his ability to use words (expression) and his ability to comprehend them (reception) – he still remains linguistically adept in many ways, particularly when responding to and talking about poetry. At such times he is noticeably concise and articulate, his comments considered, knowing and, in their own right, ingenious, even if their precise meaning sometimes eludes me.

Whatever his words mean, they are words all the same, and I share 'their associations, their public meanings'. I feel therefore that it is my failing if I don't understand him, my inability to process what, after all, are perfectly well-formed utterances. One needs to accommodate, to help recover meaning, to assume that meaning is habitually present in some form. Always. Otherwise one simply reaffirms the disease and effaces the person, missing opportunities for connection.

I'm still trying to work out exactly what I want to say about these things. There is, however, one thing of which I'm certain: the more time I spend with Robert, the more convinced I am that he retains an essential awareness, a capacity for discrimination and appreciation.

26 January 2016

This morning we had Shakespeare, Housman and Elizabeth Bishop. In between the poems we spent time looking out at the view that surrounds his top-floor apartment, picking out features in the ever-unfolding landscape: far-off farms and villages, woods and lakes, jutting steeples, the unreal power plant.

Later, just before I was about to leave – perhaps he sensed departure in my gathering of books and papers – he picked up a copy of Jacques Prévert's poems from a side table, opened it at random and, in the original French, began to read aloud. As he did so, he held the book high in one hand and, with the other, marked out metrical time, rhythmically flicking the air for emphasis. Although I struggled to follow the words, for I only have a little French, I was struck by the depth and feeling of his delivery, the subtle modulation of his voice, along with the accompanying gestures – and I saw him, forty years ago, reading aloud to and holding a classful of students, just as he was reading to and holding me now.

3 February 2016

The receptionists finally seem to know me. No longer do I have to explain to bemused-looking ears who I am and what I'm doing here. Now they anticipate me: 'Ah, yes. Robert. Take a seat', after which I wait for one of the on-call care staff to take me – via an intricate and never-ending series of stairs, landings, and corridors – up to his apartment on the second floor.

I like these brief intervals while I wait to be collected: they give me time to wander about the lobby and survey this infinitely fascinating space. The lobby is the epicentre of the retirement village, the place where its four-hundred-odd residents come to eat, drink, shop, and socialize. By no means distastefully, its main interior space, the 'village square', simulates the bright urban outdoors: through a broad skylight directly overhead light pours down on a mock streetscape of leafy trees and bushes, Edwardian street lamps, and park-style benches and tables, where people gather for morning coffee or simply sit, in the company of others, watching the world go by. Running along one side of the square is a small arcade that houses a hairdressers and beauty salon, a fitness suite (including steam room and spa pool), a laundry, a library, a crafts and woodwork room, an IT suite and greenhouse. On the other side of the square, facing the arcade, is the resident-run village shop, a café bar and restaurant, and village hall which, although used during the day for various events and activities (village meetings, luncheons), fizzes into life in the evenings when it plays host to an eclectic range of live entertainment (everything from solo vocalists to school choirs and rock and roll cover bands).

All in all, the village puts me in mind of a more leisurely Centre Parcs or tamer kind of holiday resort – a place where even the most seasoned of pleasure-seekers might spend a day or two without being unduly bored.

5 February 2016

Although meccas of positive ageing, retirement communities like the village are sometimes criticized for being closed institutions. Situated at the edge of towns and cities, snuggled away from the wider community and watched over by CCTV cameras and security personnel, they are safe, highly managed places, though free of many of the restrictions that traditional care homes place on residents. Indeed, for better or worse, it was this balance of high security and relative independence that appealed to Robert and his daughters when, after it had become clear that he was struggling to manage by himself, he moved into the village just over eight years ago. Unlike alternative forms of housing, the village afforded autonomy and self-determination, enabling him to continue enjoying a free and untrammelled life. (Rachel: 'Dad's always been a free spirit. He really has.')

Yet although village residents are free to come and go and do as they please, there are strict conditions attached to their tenancies. To preserve the utopian order of the place, covenants must be observed, house rules followed, such that any serious or recurring violation, no matter how venial or unintentional, runs the risk of eviction (a detail omitted in the sales brochures). Naturally this is something that troubles Susan and Rachel, for if Robert's behaviour 'deteriorates', he'll have to relocate to a place where, as Rachel puts it, 'he'll be locked in and won't know a single face'. They wonder how long they can keep him here, how long their complex and expensive 'jigsaw of care' will hold out.

For the moment, though, he is faring well. He is popular among the village people: they have a sincere affection for the retired academic, this richly spoken, dapper man who radiates charm and refinement. Everyone appears to know him – I note with interest how often he is hailed whenever he is down in the village centre. Women pay him particular attention, engaging him in flirty small talk or calling after him when he passes by.

He seems equally content in his own company, alone in his cosy top-floor flat. Its four rooms (kitchen, bathroom, bedroom, lounge, plus hallway) are light and well-furnished – books, naturally, being the stand out feature, books in every room, on shelves, on tables, in neat, and not so neat, piles on the floor, a library that has followed him throughout his life. Each book bears his pencil-written signature and many are annotated in his distinctive oblique. And though I suspect he can no longer hold in memory much of what he reads, his books still give him pleasure, are still a vital part of his life.

26 March 2016

'Nothing in the world can rob us of the power to say "I".' (Simone Weil)

The last words of the great satirist Jonathan Swift are said to have been (and I quote): 'I am fool.' Swift, who experienced severe cognitive deterioration in his later life, had been speaking to one of his servants and was unable to say what he wanted to say – all he could manage were these few anguished words of self-abasement. Yet, no matter what the extent of his impairment, his first-person utterance demonstrates that, grammatically at least, he was able to index himself in relation to his state of mind, suggesting he was conscious of his mental decline.

Various psychologists have argued that first-person pronouns – the use of 'I', 'me', 'myself' and so forth – stand for personhood or otherwise reference a personal self. Hence, so the argument goes, if the person with dementia uses first-person pronouns regularly and consistently, they will have 'displayed an intact self'. By this logic, Swift, despite his loss of reason, maintained a sense of personal identity right at the very end.

Since reading about Swift, I've taken an interest in Robert's pronouns – so much so that I've started to keep a mental tally of his 'Is' and 'mes'. Although

I've only kept an informal count, his use of these small unassuming words seems to be regular and varied – they appear in a range of speech acts, such as statements of intention ('I shall have to come back to that'), of conjecture ('I suppose'), and self-evaluation ('I think – I think I feel slightly ashamed of myself that I don't get going too quickly') – all of which, I feel, are testament to a facility for self-awareness.

But is to say 'I' a genuine act of self-reference? Does the use of first-person pronouns in and of themselves truly reflect selfhood? Some philosophers are doubtful. The Wittgensteinian scholar Michael Luntley, for example, puts it like this: 'a patient [with severe dementia] may have the capacity to utter sentences like, "I am thirsty" but nevertheless have lost the capacity to keep track of things in the way required to manifest the cognitive capacities constitutive of self-consciousness and self-reference'. In other words, just because someone is able to say 'I am thirsty' doesn't mean that they possess self-awareness and are able to keep track of things such as bodily states (they might in fact not be thirsty, might have forgotten that they recently had a drink). 'I am thirsty' utterances, according to Luntley, are no more indicative of self-consciousness than a laptop computer saying 'I need a mains power source' when its battery runs low.

Luntley might be right. Yet he offers no empirical evidence to demonstrate his claims. How does he know that the dementia patient's use of 'I' vocalizations is effectively meaningless, a mere reflex or miscue? Such first-person utterances might well be wrong on occasions, but even so it doesn't follow that they are without meaning or purpose. Surely they signify something? Whatever the case, one has little to lose in taking them at face value – treating them as stabs at meaning.

4 April 2016

An email from Rachel:

> Dad has just started going out of the village, which is worrying for them and us, and also something that we want to get on top of and yet help him

manage: he is a free person and wants to go out! And he actually found his way back from town. So we don't want this to become a reason for more drugs, or a reason why he has to leave. We want to try and work with the village to manage it, and for his benefit.

At what point along the dementia journey, I wonder, does the need to take a walk become pathological – suppressed by anti-psychotic medication?

6 April 2016

Although a poem I've never liked – have always found it overly sententious – I took along Kipling's 'If –' this morning. I wondered whether this popular poem, drilled into generations of schoolchildren decades ago, might release something in him.

I'd never read the poem aloud before and as I did so now, it all came back to me – the clotted syntax, the didactic, moralizing tone, all of which reading aloud only brought into sharper relief (at least with silent reading one can skim lines or skip them altogether).

After I'd finished reading the poem, I passed it to him. He'd been listening intently as I read, his gaze fixed on some indeterminate spot to the side of me, and now began to read the text for himself, smiling at the opening familiar lines and intoning the whole thing in a voice more patiently attuned to Kipling's syntax, a voice better able to traverse the knotty cluster of dependent clauses – and suddenly, despite myself, the poem came alive for me, came from somewhere else. The lines seemed to shed, so to speak, their formal burden, to communicate a rhetorical power and energy I'd never felt before, never once apprehended in the silent words on the page.

In his editorial notes on 'If –' in Kipling's *Selected Poetry*, Craig Raine argues that the poem's unflagging negotiation of its one 'impossibly encumbered sentence … demonstrates, in miniature, the possibility of achieving something genuinely difficult'.

Prior to hearing Robert read the text aloud, I would have thought the idea nothing but impressionistic nonsense.

24 April 2016

I've been reading *Iris: A Memoir*, John Bayley's biography of his wife, the novelist and philosopher Iris Murdoch. It's an intimate and often unflinching portrait of the great writer, who was diagnosed with Alzheimer's disease two years after the publication of her final novel, *Jackson's Dilemma*, at the age of seventy-seven. Like many dementia memoirs, *Iris* achieves much of its drama and pathos by emphasizing contrasts – life before and after – with all the changes in behaviour, identity and personality that attend the syndrome. And with an eminent mind such as Murdoch's, the contrasts are all the more acutely tragic: the once brilliant author now reduced to spending her days collecting dead leaves and watching the *Teletubbies*.

At the same time, Bayley is alert to and seeks continuities. Iris, we learn, remains responsive to the intimate verbal play and teasing that has long been part of their everyday discourse. She still laughs with him at their old jokes and silly soubriquets such that, Bayley feels, 'we are still part of each other'. Iris also retains an appreciation of ludic verse and rhyme. On one occasion Bayley recites a long-forgotten childhood rhyme to her and is struck by her response to it: 'Iris not only smiled – her face looked cunning and concentrated. Somewhere in the deserted areas of the brain old contacts and impulses became activated, wires joined up. A significance had revealed itself.'

On the whole, however, Bayley is reluctant to read to Iris. He tries a few chapters from *The Lord of the Rings* and *The Tale of Genji* ('two of Iris's old favourites') but finds the experience painfully frustrating, even though Iris recognizes and reacts to the texts: 'For someone who had been accustomed not so much to read books as to slip into their world as effortlessly as she slipped into a river or the sea, this laborious process of words clumping into her consciousness must have seemed a tedious irrelevance.'

I wonder what R thinks and feels when I read to him. Does he 'truly' enjoy the experience? Does he register the changes that come over him, sense the words cutting through, working on him? Or is he, as Bayley supposes Iris to be, vexed and embarrassed, the words a 'laborious procession', 'a tedious irrelevance'?

Who knows?

It is difficult to know another's mind at the best of times.

12 May 2016

Yesterday he underwent some form of cognitive assessment. By all accounts – technically at least – he performed poorly.

I suppose these tests, even in late-stage dementia (long after initial diagnosis) have their purpose, such as establishing the appropriate level of support, devising management plans and so forth. But in some respects, I can't help thinking that they do more harm than good, principally serving to maintain clinical control – that is, determining the competent from the incompetent – rather than maintain the well-being and standing of the examinee.

As with other forms of neuropsychological assessment, cognitive testing operates within a negative purview, is designed, as Oliver Sacks puts it, 'not merely to uncover, to bring out deficits but to decompose … [subjects] into functions and deficits'. Testing, moreover, is often self-fulfilling, subjecting participants to questions they cannot possibly answer or are likely to find, in the artificial, anxiety-inducing conditions of the testing environment, unduly complex and confounding. What day is it? What is your name? How long have you lived at this address? What is the name of the current prime minister?

Robert might not be able to answer such questions but, living comfortably where and how he is, does he need to? Not knowing his age last birthday or confusing Tony Blair with David Cameron (an easy mistake to make) doesn't preclude his living a meaningful life.

27 June 2016

I'm still reeling from the referendum result, the country having decided, by the margin of 3.8 per cent, to leave the European Union. As I walked to work on the morning of the result, passing through the town centre with its usually cheerful and vibrant marketplace, the atmosphere was one of emptiness rather than jubilation – strange, since most people here voted to leave. It all feels numbly apocalyptic, malignantly unreal.

My European colleagues, many of whom have been employed by the university far longer than I have, now find themselves living in a state of uncertainty – unsure whether they'll be granted indefinite leave to remain. More widely, there have been reports in the press of a spike in xenophobic attacks on EU citizens, with eastern Europeans, in particular, being subjected to horrendous verbal and physical abuse. And I fear that, because Brexit will be anything but a quick and easy process, things are only likely to get worse – antipathies will intensify, the country become increasingly polarized.

Agitation is abroad. Even the unflappably sedate aura of the village has been infected. There have been disputes among the residents. Robert is alleged to have struck a vocal Brexiteer with, appropriately enough, the *Guardian*. In the circumstances his actions seem perfectly venial, an instinctive response in a highly charged environment. 'Dad picks up on the feelings around him,' Rachel explains. 'It's never simply mindless agitation'. Still, she's understandably worried about the incident since 'this is the kind of thing that moves him towards having to leave'.

When I visit him a few days later, he is his usual warm self – endearing and chatty. Convening downstairs in the communal lobby area, we spend several hours together, talking and reading poetry. It is one of our best sessions to date.

And no one mentions Brexit.

12 July 2016

An exchange between the two of us:

K: An unusual poem that one ['Absences' by Donald Justice]. I'm not familiar with it – but I like some of the images.

R: What happens with me is I drop completely and I just read in the way that you read in which to bring in and to sow it up, put it round, put it into the … but then if something comes, something that suddenly emerges and there in some way to a surprise it's beginning to come from us or whoever.

K: Mmm.

R: Not because I don't care about them and I still, suppose this idleness, I can listen and enjoy.

K: Yes.

R: With Shakespeare – you can go on with Shakespeare forever – but you have to work hard.

K: Yes, you do.

R: But it's good and it's worth it.

M: You're fond of Shakespeare?

R: Yes.

K: 'Shall I compare thee to a summer's day / Thou art more lovely and more temperate / Rough winds do shake the darling buds of May / And summer's lease hath all too short a date' – I can't remember the rest.

R: No. And I know as I am now because it's simply that – that a sort of slight gathering and bits flittering here and there but not making a true effort and not letting the feeling come out and make it open and acceptable and then being brave enough to go the way.

…

K: And I think I mentioned D. H. Lawrence.

R: D. H. Lawrence very much because you – you have to sort of live with
      Lawrence because it's from beginning to end all the way – yes he's
      absolutely wonderful.

John Bayley likened the talk between himself and Iris to 'underwater sonar', with each of them 'bouncing pulsations off the other, and listening for an echo'. He adopts a kind of negative capability when their conversation breaks down, when he struggles to understand what she is saying. He tries to make a virtue of incomprehension, seeks to parody his own helplessness. He lets things pass.

I've also taken a leaf out of Keats's book, going along with the erratic flow of our conversation and listening out, à la Bayley, for meaningful echoes in Robert's talk. For even among the more incomprehensible stretches of discourse, there are moments of clarity: 'but you have to work hard', 'it's good and it's worth it' – statements that not only make sense in isolation but also contribute to the larger point he is trying to make: no matter how he puts things, he wants to talk, to make propositions, to develop an argument.

And there are other ways in which he is alert to the demands of interaction. He is able to manage the intricacies of turn-taking, to promote and maintain conversation (an ability which endures in late-stage dementia, but whose significance is often overlooked). But perhaps the most subtle aspect of Robert's talk – again a feature which is easy to neglect – is his use of hedging language ('a *sort of* slight gathering', 'you have to *sort of* live'). These utterances are not purposelessly vague, sense and precision running away from him, but are evidently motivated, mitigating as they do the force of what he is trying to say. Whatever their intended purpose, I see them as attempts at sense making, a desire, in short, to be understood.

And even if I don't fully understand him, if meaning breaks down completely, the impasse is never fatal – never stops me bouncing pulsations off him, without, as Keats would have it, irritably reaching after facts and reason.

19 July 2016

An update from Rachel:

> Things are OK-ish … Dad has been off again one time and had to be brought back by the police but he was fine. He's also had some incidents where he has lost his inhibition slightly … Otherwise he seems to be well.
>
> When I was last up – a week ago – we got your orange poem folder out and he read some: the Dylan Thomas [*Under Milk Wood*] opening, and some others. It was lovely.
>
> I've noticed – and Sarah [Robert's care manager] has too – that Dad's love of words and language is still very much there in strange new ways. For example, when you are out, he looks at the car number plates and assumes the letters are a word. Sometimes they are – like 'cap' – and sometimes he'll turn them into one. It's like he's looking for language and words.

5 August 2016

Even on the occasions when he's distant and withdrawn, that look of soft wariness in his eyes, I still press on, still persist with the poems. But I'm beginning to wonder whether this is the best way of proceeding, whether I should consider other approaches, find new ways in.

When I arrived at the village this morning, he was agitated and restless, constantly wandering in and out of the hallway. Again and again, I had to coax him back to his armchair in the living room, into which he would lower himself hesitantly – and only after I'd first established myself in the chair adjacent. Once seated, he was no more at ease, his hands firmly gripping the arms of the chair, as if he were about to push himself up and move off again at any moment. But as I began to read aloud, the poetry seemed to divert him, to fix him there, and after a while he relaxed his grip and reclined in his seat, giving himself over to the words entirely.

And here's the thing.

As I continued to read, I was struck by the absurdity of it all. There was something indecent about the hold the poetry had over him, its effect seemingly not so much of enchantment as of complete control: as long as I kept on reading, he continued to sit rigidly, passively, in his chair ... And it was too much (if not for him, then certainly for me).

After I'd finished reading (confining myself to no more than a few short poems), he was up and off, restless again. I wondered whether I ought to head after him and entice him back. But to follow him around the flat – an absurd prospect! So I let him be, quickly packing up my things before he returned to the living room, where he might've expected me to carry on with the bloody poetry.

As I left, I called out to him from the hallway. But there was no reply.

22 August 2016

According to 'Western' philosophical tradition, cognition is believed to be the quintessence of personhood.

But what about the body? The body plays a part. The self also exists in, and is expressed by, movement, gestures and habits: the quiet adjustment of a napkin during mealtimes, covering one's mouth when coughing or sneezing, and so on.

I see these embodied behaviours in Robert all the time. He will often initiate, for instance, what has become something of a ritual for us, a ritual we performed this very morning. While sitting at the side of me, he extends his legs, by way of initiation, to their full length. In response, I retract mine so that our feet are precisely side-by-side. And then, one at a time, he compares and contrasts his feet against mine, gauging the difference in size between them. (He's always been fascinated by my height and feet: 'That chap who comes here –' he likes to tell Rachel – 'he must be six feet six'.) This routine is usually conducted silently – what needs to be said? – but its purpose and meaning are self-evident.

Not so much thinking on, as thinking with, one's feet.

15 September 2016

All seems fine with R at the village. He is, according to Rachel, 'having a good period at the moment', both she and Susan having made some further adjustments to his care. Susan has obtained a portable GPS tracker – to support his independent walking (he continues to walk a great deal). The device has brought them both some peace of mind for it removes so much of the crisis element if he ever gets lost. 'It would be a simple question,' Rachel says, 'of telling someone where he is and they fetch him, rather than a full-on police search – which only adds more weight to him not being able to stay.'

30 September 2016

Of all the photographs on display in his living room, my favourite is a picture of him, aged 21 or thereabouts, taken on the day of his graduation. He peers over at us, this young R, as we sit and read together. He is smiling, looks happy with himself – the world outside Oxford, and all that it has to offer a talented young scholar, awaiting him.

Although he enjoyed Oxford and thrived there, the route to higher education was by no means an easy or predictable one, fraught as it was by doubts and anxieties over class and entitlement. Coming from a poor working-class background, he was the first of his family to go to university (the expectation was that, like his forebears, he would work the land). From a young age, he developed a love of words and wordplay, inherited from his grandfather, and excelled in his early years at school (he aced his exams, obtaining the highest score in the 11-plus). Pitched into an exclusively middle-class environment at grammar school, he was deeply insecure at first, ill at ease with the hierarchical mores and fraternal politics of the place, and he struggled to adjust socially and academically, though he eventually caught up with and overtook his more privileged coevals. Then it was the scholarship to Oxford – three more years of intellectual development and success – followed by a long and varied career teaching English literature at British and oriental universities (he can still speak snatches of fluent Mandarin and Japanese).

Over sixty years have passed since the picture was taken, but you'd have little difficulty picking him out in it – the same thick wavy hair, same open smile and shining eyes. But does the photograph still mean anything to him – does he still see himself in it? 'That chap was about quite a bit', he said when I drew his attention to it the other day. Was this reference to himself in the third person a sign that he saw someone else, that he no longer recognized himself?

At first, I thought so and felt I ought to correct him – 'That's you, isn't it, Robert?' – but there was clearly an archness about his remark (in keeping, no doubt, with his long-standing propensity for irony), a playfulness I failed to appreciate. For Robert has indeed been 'around quite a bit' (delicious understatement!), has known and been with himself for years. I smiled to myself, reproachfully tickled by my willingness to assume that his remark was merely the 'disease talking' rather than anything drolly intended on his part.

Maybe I'm reading too much into his words, seeking out elusive secondary meanings or meanings that aren't there at all. Yet I feel, have always felt with him, that the surface precision of his utterances betrays a wryness and acuity of thought – a sense of design and purpose that far outweighs the possibility of vagary or chance.

At any rate, I'm reluctant to admit that Robert is a stranger to himself.

21 December 2016

Much to my regret, I hadn't seen him for a while – today was my first visit since September. He didn't recognize me initially, nor seem to know why I was there. He was sluggish, indifferent, sunk deep in his armchair (he hadn't slept well, had been up and about all last night, Fiona the carer told me on the way up). But the poetry worked its magic – at length he seemed restored to himself.

In keeping with the season, I had brought along Shakespeare's 'When icicles hang by the wall' song from *Love Labour's Lost*. As he read the poem, a small, sly grin spread across his face, peaking at the refrain 'While greasy Joan doth keel the pot', which he emphasized with drawn-out throaty relish. (I later looked up 'keel' in the dictionary; its meaning was not what I expected.)

When he reached the end of the poem, stumbling slightly over the sequence of hooty vowels, 'Tu-whit; / Tu-who', he looked up at me, paused, and said, 'I got my owls mixed up.'

24 January 2017

The management at the village feel that Robert has now reached a point where, unless he receives virtually round-the-clock care, they can no longer accommodate him. His daughters, determined to maintain his independence for as long as possible, are already spending a small fortune on his care, not to mention having to coordinate the whole complex support operation, which involves them constantly having to travel up and down the country. They tell me things have become unsustainable and have little option now but to consider care home places for him, since 'the next step is approaching'.

Meanwhile, the poetry continues unabated.

23 February 2017

Storm Doris arrived yesterday, bringing rain, hard rain, and gusts of wind up to ninety-four miles per hour. I would have postponed my visit but wanted to see him, to know how he was faring on the other side of town. As I left home, the wild weather conjured, to borrow a phrase from Al Alvarez, 'all the poetic cliches' – the saplings plied double, the rooks blown about the sky.

Inside his flat, the wind pummelling the windows, it was near-impossible to talk – I thought the trembling panes would shatter at any moment. R, however, seemed unfazed – at any rate he didn't let the storm interfere with his reading, his otherwise resonant voice muffled by and barely emerging from the din.

But I couldn't focus, distracted as I was by the teetering glass – and now, suddenly, by the chairs shaking and sliding about on the balcony outside. I kept wondering whether I ought to go out and secure them or bring them inside, whether, if I didn't, he might do so himself and risk being swept over the rail. But why would he venture outside in such foul weather? He is aware of and sensitive to his surroundings.

All the same, returning home on the tram, I couldn't stop thinking about it, couldn't dispense with the image of him wandering about, Lear-like, in the storm.

12 March 2017

Sometimes I wish I could be easier with him. Sometimes I feel I'm too stiff, too gauche. I wish I had, or could replicate, the breezy naturalness of his carers, who relate to him without any apparent self-consciousness and in an entirely authentic way. I like their way with language, their sobriquets and terms of address – their 'ducks', 'chucks' and 'mateys' – which are far from condescending, are genuinely bonhomous, and which he clearly appreciates. Coming from me, such words would be marked and hollow – dead upon voicing. And so I stick to a strained semi-formality, which feels faintly repellent against their easy patter.

4 April 2017

'Whan that Aprill …'

I took along a few pages of the *General Prologue* and handed them to him, more or less without comment. He hesitated for a moment, as though considering how to begin – then pitched himself into it, switching to a sing-song voice that brought out the liquid music of Chaucer's Middle English. As he intoned the lines, it felt as though he wasn't so much decoding, reading the words off the page, as they were flowing out of him, were part of him.

It never fails.

29 June 2017

There has been an incident at the village involving R and another resident (am not certain of the details – feel it would be indelicate to ask). Rachel has been up for a few days, advocating on his behalf. 'These issues,' she writes, 'are always difficult to tackle as we only have the perspective from the "other person" since Dad cannot remember or represent himself in terms of what happened, and on-one else was there.'

6 August 2017

His propensity for portmanteau-like words. Words instinct with the sounds and meanings of other words, such as 'greep', 'crumly', and 'chumperling'. These wonderful coinages most commonly occur when he's responding to a text, commenting on its meaning or a particular stylistic feature: it's as though they provide some exegetical insight otherwise denied him by the customary resources of the language – all part of a larger effort of groping towards meaning. He often accompanies them with complementary non-verbal gestures, principally various strains and speeds of finger waggling: a fast motion for a verb, a slower, more open gesture, for other parts of speech. Although on the surface they seem nonsensical, these portmanteau words are evocative of sense – there is not only a gamey semantic quality to them but also a structural logic, comprised as they are of phonemes that harness the standard sound patterns of English.

It is not uncommon for the speech of people with dementia to be laced with neologisms and circumlocutions. In Robert's case, I don't see them as confused violations, words produced without consideration of the listener. They evidently have intended referential meaning, and even if that meaning isn't fully or immediately recoverable, one can still appreciate their sound and cadence, their Jabberwocky-like texture.

24 November 2017

An email from Rachel. I suppose it was only a matter of time.

It looks like Dad is going to be leaving when a place next comes up at the care home we have identified, and we wanted you to know. We don't know when this will be – it's all very uncertain – it could be a week, could be 10 weeks (unlikely that long but it's hard to tell). When a place does come up, we will have to move quite quickly – within 4 or 5 days to take the place.

I'm letting you know this just in case you wanted to visit Dad again in the next weeks before Christmas in case he moves …

It's only as I'm writing this I am allowing the sadness to come in because we have been so caught up in fighting it all but actually I can't let that come in and nor can Susan because we have to act, so please excuse the business-like-ness about something so huge.

Susan and I have tried every possible thing to keep Dad in his home and to keep him FREE, as this is who he is. We have a huge complex web of care making this possible. We've found solutions to his not being able to use money, to wandering, to all sorts. But it's reached a point where there aren't any solutions, other than someone living with him 24/7 which we can't afford and he would not want.

He may end up still being around until later in January as we have no idea! But you might want to visit before then if you did want to see him just in case.

11 February 2018

It's taken longer than expected, but a place at the home has finally become available. He'll be leaving at the end of the week. Rachel is up, staying with him to oversee the move.

14 February 2018

It was getting dark when I arrived at the village (almost certainly for the last time). As I made my way to the entrance, I caught sight of one of his lighted windows, stopping for a moment to look up and see if there was any movement behind it – whatever that might have signified. I thought of the opening scene in Joyce's story 'The Sisters', the young narrator peering up at the 'faintly and evenly' lit window of his old friend's house, contemplating the fateful scene within.

Rachel met me in reception, and we went up to the apartment together. On the way up she told me that he didn't understand what was happening, didn't understand the move, although she and Susan had told him a great deal about it, had done their best to prepare him. I was free, if I wanted, to say something, whatever I thought would be useful. But I didn't say anything. I didn't know what to say.

Rachel's being there made things easier, lightening what otherwise would have been a solemn evening. I loved listening to the exchanges between the two of them, their affectionate demi-banter, and felt like a gink when, somewhat officially, I produced my yellow folder of poems and proceeded to read from Tennyson's 'Ulysses':

> We are not now that strength which in old days
> Moved earth and heaven, that which we are, we are;
> One equal temper of heroic hearts,
> Made weak by time and fate, but strong in will
> To strive, to seek, to find, and not to yield.

When it was time to leave, I went over to him to say goodbye. Unsure whether to shake his hand or pat him on the shoulder, I put my hand out in a sort of indeterminate gesture between the two. He took it and held it and we shook for a while. I wished him well, said I'd be seeing him around, I was sure. Then I quickly gathered my things and headed down with Rachel to the entrance lobby, where we hugged, and I stepped out into the rainy night.

25 February 2018

By all accounts the move has gone smoothly and he is settling in well. Rachel speaks approvingly of his new abode – a 'friendly, kind and homely' place that provides excellent round-the-clock care and a stimulating, person-centred environment. He has free run of the place, is free to walk about wherever and at whatever time he likes. The staff have taken to him (how could they not?), as have his fellow residents. He doesn't want for company.

'It's early days,' Rachel writes, 'but a very good start. It is the right place, totally worth waiting for. It feels a huge relief. And it was the right moment.'

21 April 2018

Rachel asked me whether I wanted any of his books. A small number went with him, but most remain on the shelves in his apartment – there isn't space for them all in his new room. So today, a brilliant spring day, the first full day of sun since the heavy snows earlier in the month, I returned to the village and spent several hours combing through his bookshelves.

It was strange to see the old place again – almost bare, stripped of its contents bar the books and a few items of leftover furniture. Even so, as I walked around the flat, I half expected to find him in one of the empty rooms. Rachel gave me virtually free run of the shelves – except for a few books of familial significance, I was welcome to anything I wanted. (In anticipation, I'd brought along several large boxes, but now that I was here, face-to-face with his actual personal library, the prospect of filling them all seemed indecent, a violation.)

As I worked my way through the shelves, it became apparent that the books were organized in no particular fashion – weren't, as Walter Benjamin would have it, 'touched by the mild boredom of order'. Which pleased me. Disparate authors and subjects were grouped together, such that certain books turned up in unexpected places, adding to the delight of discovery: Erich Auerbach's *Mimesis* buried among volumes of Anglo-Saxon place names, Dylan Thomas's *The Collected Stories* jostling with a sequence of Japanese novels and poetry.

But the books that appealed to me most were those which he had annotated. Many were replete with various marginalia – approving comments, sceptical questions, emphatic underlinings – all of which, I thought, might reveal something of a hitherto unknown and unknowable inner life. Like all intellectuals, he evidently read with a pencil in his hand, his thoughts and musings regularly juxtaposing those of the author he was in conversation with. These were books he hadn't so much read as inhabited, and leafing through them induced in me a kind of thirst, a textual craving, my prior compunction giving way to a sudden mania, a pressing desire to ensure that I hadn't overlooked anything of significance – books of his that would let me in, in some way.

By the end of the day, I'd filled several boxes, not only my own but a few extra I'd found lying around the flat. It was, on reflection, an indecent number of books: riddled with great carious gaps, his old shelves looked rather pitiful now. But I had the books I wanted – the books that seemed to embody the course of his intellectual life, the books through which he might continue to speak in absentia.

3 May 2018

I keep thinking of poems I would have liked to have shared with him, to have heard him read. Most days I think of something. Today it was 'Naming of Parts'. Yesterday, it was Elizabeth Bishop's 'The Fish', and a few days before some of Larkin's poems. The list ramifies endlessly.

12 May 2018

'A life that has been well lived and a shared sense of happiness and accomplishment are ever after seen through the smudged glass of its last few years.' (Sherwin Nuland, 'Alzheimer's Disease')

I think many would agree with Nuland's assessment. Yet why should illness late on in life tarnish the life before? One's triumphs, achievements, feats, exploits (and everything else besides) still speak for themselves, are no less valid or authentic, no less what they were. I think we should try – to stick with Nuland's metaphor – to keep the glass clean, to bring the life back into unsullied focus, to see it for what it was, what it continues to be.

24 July 2018

This morning, as I was going through his books (all of which I've finally arranged on the shelves in my office), I found a small sheet of paper tucked inside a slim volume on Chinese history. The sheet was brown and foxed with age and stood out clearly among the clean white pages I happened to be flicking through. One side of the sheet was blank, but on the other there was a short, handwritten note. The text was undated (though it looked relatively recent) and was composed in a precise, spidery hand. It read:

> I Robert S, still working not easily, another.
>
> What loss is it to do something?
>
> Time passes.

5

The doctor as writer, the writer as doctor: A conversation with Gavin Francis

There's no need for fiction in medicine, the facts will always beat anything you can fancy.

– ARTHUR CONAN DOYLE

Gavin Francis is one of Britain's most celebrated doctor-writers. Since qualifying in medicine in 1999, he has published nine books as well as numerous articles and essays in *The Times*, the *Guardian*, the *London Review of Books*, *Granta*, and *The New York Review of Books*. He has received various awards for his writing, including the Scottish Book of the Year (2013) for *Empire Antarctica: Ice, Silence & Emperor Penguins*, an account of his time spent as base-camp doctor at a remote Antarctic research station, and the Saltire Non-Fiction Book of the Year (2015) for *Adventures in Human Being*, a cultural exploration in medicine and the human body. He is a fellow of the Royal Society of Literature, and a fellow of the Royal College of General Practitioners. He lives and practises medicine in Edinburgh, Scotland.

I interviewed Francis at the National Library of Scotland in December 2019. When we met, I was a little ruffled. Getting to Edinburgh from Nottingham had been, to put it mildly, an ordeal. Changing at Newark station, I had left one of my bags on the train – a bag containing, among other things, my voice recorder and interview questions – and had to wait several anxious hours for the train to return before I could reclaim it … But Francis immediately put me at ease – he is warm, good-humoured and disarmingly modest. He is also generous with his time – the day we met was one of his writing days, and he spent the best part of the afternoon answering and going back over my questions, never seeming to mind when, Columbo-like, I (repeatedly) asked him just one more thing.

KH: In *Adventures in Human Being* you state that when you were younger you didn't want to be a doctor. How did your interest in medicine emerge?

GF: I was interested in mapping and geography and I wanted at first to be a geographer. I came across an atlas of human anatomy – not really a kid's one but a relatively basic one, and I found it completely intoxicating and enthralling. I had always had the sense that it would be good to get a trade, some kind of sellable trade, a useful occupation that would always mean I could find work. And I wanted to travel. And so when I fell in love with this atlas of anatomy, I thought instead of being a geographer and trying to travel and make maps, why don't I become a doctor, understand this incredible topography of the body and then use that skill to travel? So that was the way round it was. When I went to medical school interviews I was very honest – I said I just want to learn all about the human body and get a really useful skill. And they seemed to think that was good enough to let me in.

KH: How do you balance your two careers? Do you see yourself more as a writer than a doctor or the other way round?

GF: I balance them by doing half the time each. So I do two and a half days a week as a doctor with some out of hours work at weekends, which probably works out at three days a week and the rest of the time I'm writing. I've got young children, so I'm at home a couple of days a week and I write while they're in school. I do most of my writing in the mornings. I find it's a really lovely balance. If I have a big deadline for a book I've got to finish, I take a week or so holiday from the GP clinic to work flat out at it. But I find it much harder to do nothing but write. It's nice to alternate.

KH: The writer Andrew Solomon describes you – along with physicians such as Henry Marsh, Atul Gawande – as being part of a new generation of doctor-writers who have undertaken to reconcile the medical/technical with the person and the personal. Would you say this is a driving element behind your writing, to bring the twin narrative of doctor and patient together?

GF: Yes, the reason I write books is because I want to articulate and communicate something of my experience, and there's no better job than medicine for giving you a synoptic, panoptic view of humanity at its most extreme moments. And if you're interested in medicine, one of the real motivations is people's stories, getting involved in people's stories, helping them in little practical ways. So it seems completely natural to me to want and try to communicate that wealth of experience in a way that people can tap into and enjoy it.

KH: Is the person foremost and the science secondary, or are the two integrated? A lot of clinical writing is dispassionate and impersonal, but I think it's fair to say that in your stories people are at the forefront.

GF: Yes I think so. If I wanted to write scientific journalism, I'd be a scientific journalist. But I'm not *that* interested in the science. I'm much more interested in the science as a use to guide optimal treatment, and as a source of wonder, or about the incredible intricacy of the human body and how it all works most of the time. So they are the kind of utilities of science for me. I could never choose just one tiny specialist area of science to devote myself to – my interests are too broad.

KH: Does being socialized in a specialized technical language make one lose sight of the person as a patient – and would you say that one of your aims is to reclaim ordinary language as a way of seeing the person?

GF: No, I don't think so. I think scientific language is a shorthand and it's used to facilitate speed of communication between peers. It's also maybe used a little bit to distance yourself from the intensity of the emotion associated with different medical conditions. I mean if you can describe it dispassionately it's less hurtful – especially concerning psychiatric diagnoses: a lot of mental health problems are basically existential crises and it's easier just to put that in dispassionate terms.

KH: I'm reminded of something you say in *Shapeshifters* – the chapter on death where you describe your experiences of shadowing a pathologist. At one point you ask her, 'You see so much death … how does it affect you?' And she replies, after a short, considered pause: 'it always makes me want to celebrate being alive'. How do you deal with being exposed to death and serious illness on a regular basis? Does the technicality of medicine, of its language, help with that?

GF: I think so, yes. When you're in a clinical meeting and you're discussing somebody who's had a terrible diagnosis – some terminal cancer diagnosis – you can talk about it very quickly and dispassionately with colleagues and they know exactly what you mean, without having to go into any elaborate detail. But I don't think that helps with coping with the death. The only thing that helps with that is having down time and breaks and space to think about it in perspective. And it's also a great privilege. It's a privileged position you occupy to be invited into people's homes at these extremes of life and death, the beginning and end of life. You're put in a position where you're welcomed into the family at these critical moments and you witness things on a weekly or monthly basis that most people only go through two or three times in a lifetime, and that feels like a great privilege but it can also get overwhelming and that's why I think we have such an enormous level of burnout in the profession. But for me, if I get enough downtime – and I've only been practising for twenty years, maybe if you ask me in another fifteen years I'll struggle more – but for me as long as you get enough off time you can process it and keep it in perspective, and those moments can … instead of becoming overwhelming or too burdensome, can become kind of inspirations to tap you on the shoulder and say, 'Are you living your life the way you're supposed to be living it? Where do you want to be living it? Are you – I mean we've got a short life, we're all going to die soon – are you doing what you want to be doing, what you should be doing? Is your life worthwhile? Do you feel you're contributing in the way you should be?' And those kind of reminders come along a lot thicker and faster for clinicians like me or district nurses who deal with this even more often than I do. So I feel mixed about it. On the one hand it is very burdensome, but on the other hand it's a great privilege if you can keep it in perspective and use it as a reminder of your own mortality.

KH: Do you find as you're becoming more experienced that your relationship with patients changes? Henry Marsh talks about how, when he was younger, he was able to distance himself from his patients, but now, towards the end of his career, he finds himself much more emotionally attuned – getting more attached to them, which he puts down to experience and ageing. I don't know if that's something you've found?

GF: Yes, interesting. As you get older you accrue a much larger archive of sad stories and disasters. So I think the longer you've been practising, the more you're aware of how badly things can go wrong. When you're younger and you've just qualified you've got a very much more of a protocol-based approach. When you're younger and you've just qualified in medicine there's a pressure to look competent, to act the part, because you don't feel the part, because you've just qualified. You

don't have a big register of experience. And so you have this pressure
to look competent, and I think this makes you a bit more mechanistic
or a bit more protocol driven. But I think as time goes on – I definitely
get better at my job as I get older, I definitely find it easier in some ways
because I'm better at it and I've seen the situations before, but I also feel
very much that your awareness of how badly things can go wrong is
much more acute. And somehow because you're not so dependent on
the whole image and the whole professionalism and the whole protocol,
you let much more of yourself come to the surface in your encounters,
which exposes you in a way. And I think that's what Henry describes
very well, because when he was at the top of his game after forty years in
his career, he doesn't need to worry about protocols or professionalism
he just *is* it – his whole body, his whole social engagement has become
incorporated by the spirit of his being a neurosurgeon, and so he's just
being himself when he's engaging with people. He's not stepping into
anything. And as you know he has stopped operating now, though he
still teaches.

KH: On to another career now with his writing.

GF: Yes – wonderful books.

KH: Does reading also help you reflect on, and come to terms with, the
        tragedy you encounter?

GF: Yes, I think so. Reading is a way of giving yourself dry runs or rehearsals
        of imagining different life situations. So for me as a way of informing
        myself – I might read Andrew Solomon for an insider's view on what it's
        like to have suicidal depression, and Kay Redfield Jamison to read about
        what it's like to have bipolar illness. So there's lots of different functions.
        If you're a bibliophile you're going to turn to books for all sort of things.

KH: One thing that comes out in your books is that you communicate
        humility – in certain instances you describe your fears, lack of
        knowledge and doubt, as though you were exposing yourself, removing

the mask, which is really refreshing. Is this something you consciously do or is it just part of the way you write and reflect on what you do?

GF: No, I think it's just part of my personality really. It's also part of being a GP, in that if your perspective in medicine is one of a GP you're never going to be an expert in anything. What you're expert at is dealing with a huge variety of things competently and knowing when you need the experts, whereas the psychological framework with which a specialist like Henry Marsh goes into a consultation is about the fact that he's a consultant specialist. So the patient is looking for mastery of the situation from them, whereas if a patient comes to me they're not looking for mastery of the situation necessarily, they're looking for an interpreter and a guide.

KH: With respect to your role as a GP, what about those patients you encounter who might not 'technically' be ill but have just lost their way in life – who are facing some kind of existential crisis – but who still come to see you? How do you deal with this as a doctor? Can medicine deal with that?

GF: It's a million-dollar question, isn't it? Essentially the question is how do we assess and gauge the authenticity of people's experience of their mental health. It's very cultural. There are some cultures where to have a nervous breakdown, and to feel that there is no purpose in your life, would not be anything to do with medicine. But we have quite a strongly medicalized culture where people who go through that feel that they – many of them feel that they – have a correctable medical condition and through the use of drugs and psychotherapy and so on they can come through it. Yet if you were to go to a profoundly religious, less economically developed community, they would frame those things in entirely religious terms – that kind of crisis.

KH: So how do you respond – it seems to me that nowadays you not only have to be a doctor but also, as it were, a priest, a counsellor, a social worker – these roles all within the scope of eight to twelve minutes or so of consultation time?

GF: Yes, absolutely. But that's what makes it so interesting. You can't do everything. Well you approach these problems, I think, just by chatting to people – that's the core of the job – and finding out what their own expectations are, what their own beliefs about themselves are. For somebody who believes they have a correctable chemical imbalance in their brain, antidepressant drugs might well cure them – there's a massive placebo effect with antidepressants. For somebody who believes that they've lost their faith in God and purpose and value and meaning of life, nobody but some kind of clergyman is going to be of benefit to them, and so each situation has to be taken on its own merits and people guided the way that's most going to benefit them. It's part again of being a GP and not being a specialist. I'm not a psychiatrist so I'm not going to tell people, 'Oh you have this. You need this.' I'm just going to try and guide them the right way.

KH: What's your attitude to social prescribing – to reading groups, gardening clubs and so on. Do you think there's a place for it, that it's effective?

GF: Yes absolutely, especially at the milder end if people are able to get out and about. But with a lot of severe mental illness people can't get out at all.

KH: Do you ever bring up literature with patients in the consultation?

GF: Occasionally, yes – if the patient is a reader, I will do, yes. Rarely fiction or poetry, although I will occasionally. Maybe you're thinking about a piece I wrote for *Aeon* ('Storyhealing') which opened with an account of a patient of mine who'd served in Afghanistan, and I suggested he read Phil Klay's book about Iraq (*Redeployment*) – short stories about Iraq. But usually it's more non-fiction. Nathan Filer wrote a wonderful book recently about schizophrenia (*The Heartland*). Some patients of mine – mostly ones who have relatives who have schizophrenia rather than being in inverted commas 'schizophrenic' themselves, I'd recommend that book to them, to try to help them understand more about this weird diagnostic label.

KH: *The Heartland* – a book very much steeped in people's stories and biographies.

GF: Yes, it goes through four or five case studies and shows how this diagnostic label became attached to this person, and how there might be other ways of thinking about the psychotic experience they had.

KH: It's very much a literary book, I would argue, rather than explicit self-help book. Is there a sense that literary texts work differently than cognitive behavioural therapy books?

GF: Yes, it's different stories. Depends whether someone engages better with that kind of storytelling rather than a 'how to' manual.

KH: You have a particular facility for describing the human body in terms of other entities – landscape and the natural world in particular. Indeed, one could argue that *Adventures in Human Being* is a kind of extended metaphor. Do you think in metaphor naturally with respect to medicine and the body? How does it (metaphor) influence the way you write about and respond to patients?

GF: It's a tricky question. I mean I think in metaphor when I'm writing, of course, to find the best way to try to communicate a particular situation or describe an encounter or describe some aspect of the physical universe: whether it's somebody's knee or whether it's somebody's facial expression or whatever. So I think in metaphor and I write in metaphor. I don't know – I've never thought about it in terms of my patient encounters. When you're examining people – certainly in a physical illness rather than a mental illness – you use this quite rigid framework you're taught at medical school, which is very useful because it's translatable and it's reproducible, and that's how you describe things: you describe a joint in terms of whether it's got an infusion, whether it's red, whether it's got crepitus; you describe lungs in terms of whether they've got bronchial breathing or crepitations within them. So there's a rigid framework there which you're already tapping into.

KH: Do you think that's where it comes from then – your enthusiasm for metaphor? Your writing is shot through with vivid figures of speech, which makes readers see things in a different way.

GF: Yes, I'm trying to – the purpose of a good one is to make the reader think about something in a new way. I mean there are a load of metaphors which have just become clichés, part of normal everyday speech and don't arouse any interest whatsoever – they're not going to make you wake up and take notice.

KH: Do you think being a writer makes you a better doctor?

GF: Yes, I think so. It definitely makes me more reflective. It makes me more aware of the value of story, the value of choice of words, the careful choice of words. It makes you better at rapid assessment of a situation. It makes you better at delivering a synopsis or a story back to the patient which they can take on and make their own. A lot of my job is interpreting symptoms, making a diagnosis and then selling that diagnosis back to the patient, with the reassurance that I've seen this before and that you're part of this group of people who have this thing and this is how one gets better from it.

KH: The doctor-writer Theodore Dalrymple writes somewhere that though he would like his doctor to be cultured rather than a philistine, he would like them even more to have a grasp of physiology and biochemistry, as if he were poo-pooing the idea that it doesn't really matter how well-read you are.

GF: I think that's true, because what you don't want is a doctor that doesn't know what they're talking about with the physical things. It's all very well to be well up on your medical humanities but if you can't actually make accurate diagnoses and formulate plans of therapy, then you shouldn't be in the job.

KH: Does narrative and having an awareness of other people's lives help you to do that more competently?

GF: Yes – I don't think the two are necessarily easily extricable. There are different kinds of doctors, aren't there? There's that lovely paragraph in John Berger's book *A Fortunate Man*, where he talks about different kinds of doctors. He says there are doctors who are businessmen; there are doctors who are scientists; there are doctors who are healers; there are doctors who are priests. And it's true and if you look at a big group practice with lots of doctors, you'll find that patients gravitate to different kinds of doctors depending on what they want and what they think they need at that time.

KH: Do you play different doctor roles depending on the patient?

GF: Yes, very much. I work in a small practice so people don't have much choice. And I've said before that I think the very best doctors are the ones who can accurately figure out very quickly what kind of doctor the patient needs, because you're far more likely to get better if you're getting the advice, or being engaged with in the way that you hoped you would be.

KH: In relation to different roles, how much of you – your self – does your own character come into other people's stories? How do you craft yourself into your writing?

GF: I try to adopt a style which is what I would most enjoy reading. So I try not to have too much 'I', 'I', 'I' – 'I did this.' 'I did that.' 'I thought about that.' Kathleen Jamie writes beautifully about this: she writes a first draft and then she goes and crosses out everything that begins with 'I'. So, it's really just what kind of writing you like to read, isn't it? So I don't like a lot of 'I', 'I', 'I' and so will try to pare that back if starts to creep in.

KH: As a way of giving people their voices and letting their experiences come through, you sort of suppress your own a bit?

GF: Yes, absolutely. That old adage 'show don't tell' – you try and allow people to let the image that you're building tell the story, rather than explicitly articulating everything.

KH: You have a sharp eye for detail – details that most people would overlook. Would you say you've been socialized into detail through writing and reading or would you say you were naturally observant?

GF: I think you're talking again about the pathology essay in *Shapeshifters*. No – it just comes naturally to describe things in those terms. It's much more vivid to say that 'the gallbladder feels like a bag of dice' – doesn't it? – than 'the gallbladder felt lumpy with bits of grit'?

KH: Regarding narrative description, how do you handle clinical anecdotes in your writing? I'm thinking here when it comes to anonymization, and respecting confidentiality, and changing details, what counts as fiction and non-fiction?

GF: That's a big grey zone. These are not scientific case studies. They're not published in *The Lancet*, so there's a lot that's modified and changed to make sure that nobody could recognize anything. There's only a couple of stories in *Shapeshifters* that were so vividly unusual that they could probably be traced back, and in both those cases I actually spoke to the patient involved, and it was fine. But I have to take it case-by-case and I nearly always feel that that puts too much pressure on the patient to agree if they want to, and it's much safer, both for them and for me, just to modify all the critical details. These are just GP consultations and experiences in Accident and Emergency. These are all things that happen all the time. It's not like I'm writing science fiction. So everything that's in there has actually happened.

KH: Nonetheless, I would suggest you have a novelist's eye, novelist's way of looking at things.

GF: You mention the novel – novelists steal hugely from real life all the time.

KH: I read somewhere that Conrad said he didn't have the imagination to invent his characters – they were all real, taken from his seafaring experiences.

GF: So I think, yes, novelists stand on a borderline between the real world, and their fictional creations, and I'm standing in a similar place but with a different focus. Because I have to fictionalize enough of the details to make it – just to make it safe for me and the patient. I feel entirely relaxed about how much has been changed in order to make it safe for me and my patients. But I'm aware that some of my readers feel that with a non-fiction book you have a contract with the reader, that everything has to be just as it is, and so I'm very up front. That's why the very first page of *all* of my books that touch on medicine is a note on confidentiality. I want that to be the first thing that readers encounter.

KH: Even so, I suppose you're still presented with information that can be looked at from different points of view, which in itself is an act of creation, and people have argued that even an autobiography is a work of fiction in that it's constructed from a particular point of view.

GF: Hugely. Autobiography is the genre which has got the least rules. People can do what they like with their own story. Everything's justified. That's another Berger quote – I'm sure Berger said somewhere that the logic of autobiography is that you can do whatever the hell you want.

KH: Have you ever felt inclined to write a novel?

GF: No never. Doesn't interest me.

KH: Why's that?

GF: It's just I don't feel it's what I want to get out of writing. It's a grey enough zone for me being able to fictionalize certain stories to make certain points – it's a completely different prospect writing a novel. A novel is in some ways much freer, in other ways it's much, much more constrained.

It has to have certain narrative arcs and progressions in order to work, in a way that non-fiction doesn't have to have.

KH: Just going back to Berger, because you met Berger. That must have been tremendous.

GF: Yes, a lovely, lovely man. It was a great honour to meet him.

KH: How does it feel bringing Berger's book *A Fortunate Man* to life? That's down to you – its being re-released again, brought back from the dead.

GF: I wrote to him wanting to quote him, in the eye chapter in *Adventures in Human Being*. I sent him a letter on headed note paper and it had my phone number on it, and I was at home one day looking after the kids – it was a Saturday morning, I was trying to clean the kitchen – and the phone went and this voice said, 'It's John Berger here!' And I said [simulating a surprised, awestruck voice], 'Hello, Mr Berger!' It was lovely. And we started chatting. We had a nice conversation. And spoke about *A Fortunate Man*. I said, 'Ah you know *Fortunate Man* is so amazing –' and I don't think I'd even asked to quote from *A Fortunate Man* – no that it was it: the eye chapter of *Adventures in Human Being* had a quote from his little book that he did about his cataracts (*Cataract: Some Notes After Having a Cataract Removed*).

KH: … The book with the lovely illustrations.

GF: Yes. – So we just stayed in touch. And I was going to France for some reason and he said come and stay, and so I went to visit him. I said I'd love to get this (*A Fortunate Man*) back into print. Do you mind if I ask around? And he said, 'Carry on! Whatever you like!'

KH: Did you learn much from him, then, as a writer and a doctor, from *A Fortunate Man*?

GF: From that book I think – it's emblematic of a principle in writing: just do what you really want to do. Don't try to follow some pre-set guide of idea of genre, or idea of approach, or idea of length of a book or how a book should look. That ultimately is the publisher's decision. My work as a writer is to produce the book I most want to produce and then go to the publisher and say, 'Do you like this? Is it worth publishing?' And that's what I learned from Berger: that he could do that. His books are incredibly eclectic, and it's because each time he had a different vision of what the book was going to be like.

KH: And that's been liberating for you.

GF: Yes, think so, yes. The book I've got coming out in May about islands and isolation (*Island Dreams*) is very different from anything I've done before. It's quite short, it's very digressive, allusive, it's like a confessional essay in some ways, all interspersed with old maps. It examines the allure of the idea of being on a desert island from all kinds of different angles – and I would never have done that if I hadn't felt so liberated.

KH: Do you generally find writing liberating, and if so, from what?

GF: No, not liberating. I find it satisfying. I find I get a lot of meaning out of it and a lot of worth. I enjoy it. A lot of writers hate writing, and I always feel, well, don't do it.

KH: You've always said that for you it comes fairly easily.

GF: Yes, I just enjoy it. I enjoy trying to make a sentence. And I'm not a poet. I'm not working within that very different framework of reference. I'm just writing, I hope, good prose, literary prose, which can use, borrow, things from poetry in terms of metaphor and so on, but is still trying to drive a really clear narrative.

KH: There's a lot of research that talks about how writing is therapeutic, how, for example, keeping a diary can help maintain one's mental, and physical, well-being. Do you find writing therapeutic?

GF: Yes, I find it very – because I'm only working – I work a day in the clinic and then a day writing and then a day in the clinic again. So I find very much that my clinic days are fantastic: they're really full, busy, and you're using your brain in a very satisfying way intellectually, very engaged, but it's also exhausting, whereas sitting in silence for six or seven hours trying to write a thousand words of really clear, crisp, communicative prose uses your brain in a completely different way. So rather than therapeutic or liberating I would just say it's a kind of rebalancing. I find medicine tires out my brain in one way, and writing tires out my brain in a different way, but the two ways kind of mutually redress one another.

KH: Have you always written regularly then? Do you keep a diary as such?

GF: Yes, yes, much less now though because I write so much, but before I wrote I kept a diary.

KH: In terms of your writing a story about a patient, how would that happen? Do you think of interesting cases and take it from there?

GF: Yes, I'll start off with a theme and then I'll just think of the most illustrative examples. So with *Shapeshifters* I'd start with the theme, say, of hallucinations – psychotic hallucinations and LSD – and I would just sit and think about a patient I once knew who had a terrible time with LSD and think that's a really interesting example of how fine the line is between LSD hallucinations and a schizophrenic psychotic hallucination. And I would start writing about that – set the scene, give a bit of the basic science for the reader.

KH: Do you ever think about, as it were, writing when you're in the midst of doing something, when, say, you're with a patient? I often do and feel I have to make a note of it there and then. Are you struck by the possibilities of stories all the time?

GF: No, when I'm in the throes of a busy clinic, I'm just thinking about doing my clinic work, to the best of my ability.

KH: So the writer's side doesn't it come into it as such?

GF: Doesn't keep intruding, no.

6

April notebook: A death in the family

The grief of losing a brother or sister is the least acknowledged of bereavements within the immediate family. For how can the grief of a sibling take center stage? The parents own this grief – it belongs to them.

– DOROTHY P. HOLINGER

On 21 July 2021, my brother was diagnosed, quite unexpectedly, with terminal lung cancer (later discovered to be metastatic melanoma). He died eight months later, on 21 April 2022, at the age of forty-eight.

For reasons not immediately clear to me – a vague belief, perhaps, that this was something I should be doing at a time like this – I began to keep a notebook. Initially, I didn't have the patience or concentration to write anything except short half-formed thoughts and fragments (at times, it was all I could do to jot down a word or a phrase). But over time the entries became a little more limber, a little more expansive. I found that the simple act of writing ('the sad mechanic exercise') was a kind of numbing distraction, an act of self-regulation. I became convinced, moreover, that writing things down might, in the words of Edwidge Danticat, lead me 'to some still undiscovered and undefined "other side"', not a place of closure as such, but a place where I might at least come to some sort of acceptance and understanding.

April 21

Spend the first night at Mum and Dad's, sleeping in my old bedroom (Mum sleeps in his room – hear her weeping through the thin wall between us). I sleep fitfully, waking at 4:00 a.m. to the insufferable cooing of doves in the eaves.

How do they endure this taunting chorus every morning?

April 22

His fortitude.

April 23

The flowers start to arrive. And the cards. The endless cards …

Attempt, and fail, to make a passable poem out of their platitudes of sympathy (provisional title: 'Sincerely Speaking'):

> We wanted to reach out,
> to share our sincere condolences.
> Our sincere sympathies,
> our deepest most sincere sympathies,
> sincerely go out to you,
> to you and your family.
>
> And our hearts,
> our sincere hearts,
> our most sincere hearts,
> go out,
> sincerely go out,
> to you and your family.
>
> With warm thoughts and care,
> our sincere sympathies extend to you.
> No warm words can sincerely express

our sincere condolences,

our sincerest sympathies,

to you and your family.

April 24

(Around 1:00 a.m.)

Pull up outside the funeral parlour in the village shopping precinct.

Think of him lying inside, right next door to The Moghul* (The Moghul! The Moghul, C!)

April 26

As I step out on to the Beeston streets this morning, all red-eyed and weepy, a few lines from *Under Milk Wood* pop into my head:

Look … Captain Cat is crying

He's crying all over his nose

He's got a nose like strawberries

And rather than hide my suffering as passers-by approach, I let it come over me – make a show of my fierce tears.

Oh, my dead dear!

April 27

Void.

April 28

Momentary relief in certain actions, such as throwing a ball, rubbing an ear, scratching my face. During these micro-second moments, he's out of mind – and the laceration stops.

---

* The takeaway we used to use every Friday when we were both living at home. Each week was always the same. Him: chicken karahi (first separating the chicken from the karahi sauce to enhance the protein-to-fat ratio); me: vegetable rogan josh – which we would eat on our laps while watching Robot Wars.

The thing to do, I suppose, is to throw and scratch more often.

Continuous stream of throwing and scratching.

May 1

How can I step into May (to borrow a conceit) while you forever remain in April?

May 2

A warm spring day – I go for a run – the first in a long time. When I get back, I flop on the sofa and let the dog lick the sweat off my face.

I know she's after the salt, but it feels like a blessing all the same.

May 3

Is it now a matter of having to learn to live what the novelist David Grossman refers to as 'the inverse of life'?

May 4

'It is well known that mourners often get the illness which led to the death of a close person.' (Lily Pincus)

Visit the GP this morning to have a growth on the side of my face examined.

'I would have left it', I tell the doctor. 'But things as they are, you know – in the current circumstances …'

When, after a very quick examination, she happily informs me that it's just a wart, all perfectly benign, nothing to worry about, I feel not so much relief as mild disappointment.

As though I'd let you down.

May 6

In my discourse seminars, I always encourage students to watch out for, among other things, lists of three. Three, I tell them, is the magic number; signifies a wholesome roundness, completeness.

So when you broke the news to me – which at first I (insistently, insistently) took for one of your more outrageous practical jokes – it wasn't so much the words 'terminal' and 'months' that stood out as you saying that it was in your 'lungs, liver, and spine'.

May 11

Sit in his room for a while, attempting to parse the stillness, a stillness, it seems, that 'no power on earth can waken'.

May 12

Whenever Mum's phone pings, Dad pipes expectantly – 'Your phone's just gone, love!' – as though this could be it, the message they've been waiting for these last few weeks …

The text finally confirming that it's all been a horrible mistake.

May 13

I pick at – for reading is difficult, though read I must – the well-known mourning texts: C. S. Lewis's *A Grief Observed*, Joan Didion's *The Year of Magical Thinking*, Elisabeth Kübler-Ross's *On Death and Dying*, all of which are useful.

But the book that affects me most powerfully is Roland Barthes's *Mourning Diary* – a journal Barthes kept following the death of his mother, Henriette, to whom he was utterly devoted. It's an extraordinary book, by turns astute and desperate, the author continually off-guard, beguilingly exposed. The customary literary perception is still there, but the most interesting and moving passages are those when the great critic attempts to describe, with no hope of intellectualizing, the fallout of losing the person he loved most in the world:

> Snow, a real snowstorm over Paris; strange. I tell myself, and suffer for it: she will never again be here to see it, or for me to describe it for her.

May 14

My worst moments are at the kitchen sink.

May 15

Moving aimlessly from room to room serves a purpose, if only for the mild act of volition it compels.

How many hours has it taken me to eke out that one sentence?

Agony.

Best not to do it at all.

May 16

Ceaseless fluttering in the stomach. Sobbing. Followed by breathlessness (from suppression of sobs). Then sobbing again. Then breathlessness …

Compelling cycle of incapacity.

May 17

I should say more.

May 18

Piercing screeches overhead.

I look up and see them – the familiar sickle shapes. Swifts. Dozens of them. They're back again, which, to paraphrase Ted Hughes, means the world's still working.

It's the first time I've seen the sky in ages.

May 19

The funeral.

May 20

Whenever I drive around and see people going about their business, I'm struck by nothing more than the simple fact of their existence, their very (extraordinary) *aliveness*.

To the man over there on his bicycle: 'You're alive!' I say. To the couple sat at the bus stop: 'How do you do it?'

May 21

The cheesy 1990s pop song he used to play over and over (Haddaway's 'What is Love'). I used to rib him about it, ridicule its trite sentiments and infernal refrain. (Growing up, we never liked the same songs.)

But when I happen to hear it on the radio this morning, it sets me off like a baby.

Later on, I look it up online and listen to it over and over, finally beginning to appreciate your exquisite taste in music.

May 22

Yes, yes, life goes on. Of course it goes on. We all know that. But I can't accept that it does. Failing that, I want other people to feel something of what I feel, to know what it's like. I resent the way everyone else goes about their busy little lives – the guffawing cyclists streaming past, the ecstatically gesticulating diners in the tapas bar.

I know that we inhabit two separate worlds, you and I, and that I can't blame you for revelling in 'the stable banality of routine living.' But as you tuck into your gambas pil pil and tempura seabass (and by all means carry on: laying off won't bring him back), you should at least know that he's dead, that I'll never see him again.

May 23

At first, I baulked at all the comforting fictions. *Nanna's looking after him ... He's up there having a drink with so-and-so ...* Do they really believe these silly conceits?

But when I catch my daughter addressing the sky one evening ('Hello, Uncle Clive. How are you, Uncle Clive? – Daddy, Uncle Clive says he's with Great-Grandpa and he's having a lovely time!') I find myself colluding in the fantasy. 'That's nice,' I say. 'What's he doing?' 'He's having a milkshake and doing pull-ups.'

These exchanges – and subsequent others like them – do not presume that Uncle-Brother is still alive, only that in no way has he ceased to exist.

May 24

This morning I note the slight crack above the bathroom sink. The other week it was a scuff on the sideboard.

– Both of no consequence at all, except for the fact that the last time I saw them, he was still alive.

May 25

Not much depth to these jottings.

Still, they serve a purpose, if only to force me to think and see a bit more, to gain some purchase on the world.

May 26

As time passes, they say it gets easier, that you learn to live with it, to live without them.

But as Barthes suggests, does being able to live without someone you loved mean you loved them less than you thought you did?

May 28

If I can live a little better, embrace, say, some of his froideur, his breezy devil-may-care attitude to everything, then perhaps, perhaps …

Perhaps what? His relatively short life won't have been in vain? His suffering and death will have been worth it?

May 29

Nothing to report.

(There's nothing intrinsically interesting about death and grief.)

May 30

In the park.

If I pitch it right, get the line and length right, the ball strikes the lime tree at the bottom of the incline – such that it veers off satisfyingly out of sight, the dog scampering after it.

June 1

Great sense of sadness this morning. Denial too (he's just gone away for a while, will fetch up at Mum and Dad's today for Sunday dinner as he always does, the old litter-strewn Kia parked outside, tight against the kerb). Absurd of course. But on one level, at least, I half believe it.

June 3

Keep seeing him in crowds. He always stands out in crowds, my brother.

Managed to get up close to him the other day. Followed him down the street for a while, followed that slow, sway-rolling gait all the way from John Kirk Hi-Fi to the Beeston Bed Centre, and when he happened to turn around – sure enough, sure enough – it was him! It was him! Yes, it was!

… Except it wasn't him. (How it could it be? How could it not be?)

Disappointed, I nearly asked him if, by way of consolation, he could be my brother, pretend to be him for a while, if only for a moment. Clive. Clive was his name. He was a police officer and was big, very big, just like you. Used to mix up protein shakes in the cinema. Dog lover too … Yes, yes, I know it's a funny thing to ask – all the more so asked of a stranger – but do play along with me, humour a grief-stricken sibling anguishing in the depths of despair.

It would mean everything – something – to me.

June 4

When did it begin?

Was it there back then – the first time we'd seen each other for months – when we met at Chiquitos just over five years ago? You had just met J (who would do so much for you) and started work at the airport, a cushy post that would see you through until retirement. Things were beginning to turn around. We clinked glasses and shared a giant combo starter (nachos, chicken wings, halloumi fries).

Was it there in June 2019 when we were in Southampton for Mum and Dad's golden wedding anniversary? You spent the morning scouring the city for a gym to work out in, fetching up later with your customary protein shake and bunch of bananas. I couldn't compete for attention – the cousins, nephews, and nieces all adored you. You were the main event, the star attraction, disappearing not long after you arrived. (Always the sense with you that you had to be somewhere else, were always on the move … Where did you go, my lovely? To which quests were you yoked?)

Was it there in December 2020 when we celebrated my daughter Mae's seventh birthday, sipping prosecco in freezing Highfields Park? We kicked a football about, you with a chicken sandwich in your hand, remarking, as you sliced the ball and sent it breezing off towards the car park, 'I've still got it.' Later you mentioned that you'd been feeling unusually tired, but thought little of it, putting your fatigue down to longer shifts and overtraining.

And was it *really* there on that beautiful blue day last July, that dreadful day, the day of the diagnosis, when we were all gathered in the garden at Mum and Dad's, and Dad, speaking for everyone, even for those of us who knew something about these things, said, 'Look at him, look at him – look at the bloody size of him – and they say he's got cancer!'?

June 6

First day without tears, seven weeks after his death.

Is this too soon? (What do the books say?)

Or is this the first green shoot, the first sign of what psychiatrists call 'uncomplicated grief' or 'normal bereavement' and hence all's on track?

June 7

The thing about your death – just how exquisite it is!

Forty-eight years, in some respects, is such a perfect age to die. Presumptuous, yes. But therein rests the perfection.

June 8

You'll be stronger once you come out the other side, friends say.

Although well-intentioned, chivvying remarks of this kind ring hollow to me. Grieving (by all accounts) is never a cleanly restorative process, a discrete transition from dark night to bright day.

Julian Barnes puts it well:

> You don't come out of it like a train coming out of a tunnel, bursting through the downs into sunshine and that swift rattling descent to the Channel … you come out of it as a gull comes out of an oil slick; you are tarred and feathered for life.

Three months later, I don't feel any stronger. On the contrary, a kind of stubborn malaise, a ticklish indolence, continues to take hold. I struggle to find foot holes in the day. I let things stack up, leave things undone. I wear the same shirt over and over (what does it matter that my shirts are dirty?) and eat little except for buttered toast. The dog walks me to the park, where I moon about in the shade of the giant oak tree.

June 9

Read about Arthur Conan Doyle's attempts to commune with the dead in Edward Parnell's moving memoir of grief, *Ghostland*.

Doyle turned to Spiritualism, Parnell relates, following the death of his oldest son Kingsley, who died after being injured at the Battle of the Somme during World War I. Like so many other people who lost family during the 'Great War', Doyle attempted to contact his beloved dead, publishing in 1927 a series of 'comforting messages received from the other realm' by his wife Jean, a self-avowed medium.

During one séance, Doyle's snake-obsessed son Denis asked Kingsley: 'Where are the snakes with you?' To which 'Kingsley' replied: 'In their own place, old chap. We are so proud of you, Denis, and the way you are developing in every way.'

It is hard to credit, writes Parnell, that the creator of the uber-rationalist Sherlock Holmes so readily took these vague and banal remarks 'as solid evidence of an afterlife, and not as the understandable attempts (either consciously or unconsciously) of his wife – who had also lost her brother during the Great War – to bring comfort to a grieving old man and his family'.

But oh, the willingness to believe, Edward! The comfort of delusion!

Six hours after my brother's death, suddenly feeling the need to eat, I picked up a vegetable rogan josh from the local takeaway. Inside the foil tray, incongruous among the finely chopped carrots and onions, were six whole, ping pong ball-sized Brussels sprouts (sprouts: your absolute favourite vegetable).

It's him! Mum cried. And there and then, I believed it too. (For who else would have put them there? 'No, no, we don't put Brussels sprouts in our dishes', said the bemused restaurant owner when I phoned him the following day.)

But if you can reach us, why do it through humble brassica? Surely there's more wonderful ways of returning, more emphatic ways of letting us know?

Then again, why shouldn't you introduce yourself in such a quotidian fashion? After all, isn't that the way the dead come back to us? 'Not in the darkened rooms / Of rattling tambourines and butter muslin', as the poet Roy Fuller puts it. 'But as you boil an egg or make the bed …'

June 10

I need some clever philosophical argument, some winning conceit that justifies it all. Something from the great Marcus Aurelius perhaps, him of the crisp stoical logic.

Death, he says, is no big deal: it's simply the loss of the present moment.

Yes, that should do it.

June 11

What explanation other than the chef, having run out of the usual ingredients, reached for whatever else happened to be at hand, in this instance, Brussels sprouts, a vegetable not only not mentioned anywhere on the menu but also completely out of season at this time of year, and tossed them into the mix without so much as slicing or making the least attempt to integrate them into the rest of the dish – six huge green sprouts resting discrepantly on a bed of thin red sauce?

Any more plausible than you having something to do with it?

June 12

Question of social etiquette.

When does one stop talking about him? At what point does he rightfully slip down the conversational agenda? As far as I'm concerned, he's still the main subject of conversation (with myself).

But with other people – I see it in their faces, their forestalling gestures, the angst in their eyes – 'Don't go there', they seem to say. 'He's no longer news.'

June 13

The family playing cricket in the park, the girl hitting the ball high into the air, everyone else underneath it, waiting …

… You socking that outrageous six – the ball struck so hard ('caveman style', you called it) that you didn't bother to run – not that you could run, you and your stifling bulk, and all dressed in your tight-stripy gym gear, instead of the requisite whites (opposing team captain: 'Look at him, look at him! – He's not even dressed right!') – and all the fielders gathered on the boundary, teetering, Laurel-and-Hardy-like, beneath it, waiting … Where is it? Where did it go? It doesn't seem to be coming down, does it? Nothing up there but swifts … But it does come down, as everything must, down, right down, down through their fingers, thump down on the other side of the boundary.

Six!

June 14

Read Julia Darling's poem, 'A Waiting Room in August'.

> Acute ears listen for
> the call of our names
> across the room of
> green chairs and walls …

And, inevitably, I picture you in your green chair, waiting for one of your endless appointments, listening out for your name to be called.

When was the last time, I wonder, you heard 'those dear consonants and syllables'?

June 15

Your fifty-fifth day dead.

Impressive.

You're getting good at this.

June 17

Inadvertently catch sight of him high up on the living room shelf – and am rendered breathless for a moment.

Have to gather myself.

From now on: the need to exercise greater caution about the house.

June 18

Since I had the courtesy to let you go first, you could at least tell me something about it.

What's it like to die? How is the death?

June 20

Bump into M. in the high street. (We haven't seen each other for over two years.)

Without any phatic preamble, she launches into a litany of personal complaint – the undiagnosed tingling in the forearm, the exorbitant school fees, the cancelled flight to Dubai … (Throughout all this, silently to myself: isn't mine the bigger news, the greater grief?)

When it's my turn – time for the showstopper – I don't have the heart to upstage her.

I'm fine, I say, making my excuses.

June 21

(Late evening)

Sullen dog walk through the town centre.

Cheered on my way back by the display in the tanning store window – debonair model basking in the kindly, melanomic glow of a UV lamp.

June 23

It took me six or seven attempts to leave you after you died (you dead!). It wasn't a matter of not being able to say goodbye. Rather, each time I left the room, I just couldn't walk away with that final image of you, with how I last saw you. I would have to go back and look at you again, this time, each time, from another angle or position – from the side, more obliquely, with my eyes half-closed, squinting, or through my fingers – any view that rendered you more my brother than my brother's body. So long as I got that last look right, I reckoned, you would never be an exclusively dead person.

June 24

Why is there no serviceable 'dying language', no effective lexicon for approaching dying and death? How many times have I had to skirt the subject or resort to specious arguments and mollifying conceits?

I recall, for instance, picking you up from the hospice, and the (unusually awkward) silence in the car once our familiar prattle had dried up. You said – though not in a self-regarding way – that you felt weak, inferior. I tried to make you feel better, told you about the philosopher Wittgenstein and how he signed up to fight in the First World War, how he believed that suffering hardship and facing death would improve him, consecrate him, make him more alive.

And what's your point? you said.

Well, you know …

What was my point?

June 25

Still scan each face I pass …

Just to make sure.

June 27

Finally bring myself to check my emails.

Overflowing, pullulating inbox (endless queries, confirmations, requests).

Where does one begin?

(Barthes: 'no sooner has she departed than the world deafens me with its *continuance*.')

June 28

Food was everything to you.

You thought nothing of cracking a dozen raw eggs into a glass – then downing the lot in one long gulp.

The lengths you went to maintain that engine of yours!

Food.

Later, it became your thread of continuity, your passport to the kingdom of the well, to the life before. (You measured everything in terms of appetite – what you were eating and what you could eat.)

Stacks of it everywhere, on every surface, all within reach around your bedside – sandwiches, cookies, smoothies, pancakes, flapjacks, Yops, yoghurts, milkshakes, Müller Rices, protein bars, protein drinks, Dairy Milks, and bananas (bananas, always bananas).

Visiting you, I quipped, not very funnily, was like taking a trip to the supermarket.

Even when your appetite failed you, when you could barely eat a thing, you still wanted it near you, the sweet stuff especially.

The way you set about that bowl of Cornish ice cream, the old flicker in your eyes, the bright light returning.

June 29

I say there's no dying language, but that's not true. Or if it is true, it doesn't, shouldn't, preclude us from trying to make meaning, to express the inexpressible. Surely the attempt's the thing.

It's a point that Denise Riley makes beautifully in *Time Lived, Without Its Flow*, a linguistic and philosophical reflection on the death of her son, Jacob. The vocabulary of loss might well be wanting – there are, she observes, no specific terms for a grieving parent (or for that matter a grieving sibling) – but to concede that being in grief is incommunicable is only to 'isolate you further, when coming so close to your child's death is already quite solitary enough'.

For all its inadequacies, language offers us a way of approaching and reanimating the dead. The simplest act of predication ('He is dead') induces 'a curious linguistic quasi-resurrection', keeping alive the possibility of discussing the deceased. 'No subject,' she continues, 'can easily be conceived as extinguished, because language itself doesn't want to allow that thought; its trajectory is always to lean forward, to push it along, to propel the dead onward among the living.'

June 30

What distracts (saves?) me during the burial service is, absurdly, thinking about absurdist fiction – specifically, that preposterously droll bit in Beckett about bananas tasting sweeter when consumed on a tombstone.

July 1

I don't hear him in the trees or see him glinting on the snow (à la Mary Elizabeth Frye).

All the same, one consequence of his disappearance has been to leave me more open to mystery. No corresponding loss of faith in science and reason – I continue to love those things – but a marked susceptibility to the vaguely numinous.

My fixation, for instance, with the 'no final goodbye' scene in *Nomadland*, which I play over and over and in doing so almost begin to believe it.

'I can look down the road and be certain in my heart that I'll see my son again …'

If that doesn't work out, I'll settle for the kind of reunion that Denise Riley describes in *Time Lived Without Its Flow*.

'My best hope's to have a hallucination of his presence when I'm dying myself.'

July 3

You never cared much for literature. I could never break through, never get you into books I thought would do you good.

But you liked the Lawrence poem I showed you – applauded its sentiments at least.

I never saw a wild thing
sorry for itself.
A small bird will drop frozen dead from a bough
without ever having felt sorry for itself.

Whether these lines continued to mean anything as things got worse, I can only guess at.

But I never once recall you showing any self-pity.

July 5

The anguish continues – I suffer still – but there's a featureless intensity to it now, a persistent evenness – less C. S. Lewis's 'red hot jab' than Coleridge's 'grief without a pang'.

July 6

I remember, many years ago, reading a letter Philip Larkin wrote to the poet Douglas Dunn (1 March 1985). Larkin had recently read Dunn's volume of poems, *Elegies*, a tribute to his late wife Lesley, who died of cancer in 1981. I particularly remember the sentence – 'you have gone so far beyond me in suffering that I'm at a loss to say very much' – and I remember how taken I was by it, how I thought about it constantly, trying to imagine the scale of suffering to which Larkin alluded. Even though I hadn't read *Elegies* at the time, that sentence alone somehow conveyed the extremity, the sheer totality, of Dunn's suffering, a sense of suffering that not even the actual book, Dunn's own personal account of his pain, could convey.

I only mention this because I can't help asking the question – absurd and self-regarding though it is – what would Larkin have made of *my* suffering?

How does it compare, Philip?

How am I doing?

July 8

A few weeks before you died, I would lie awake at night wondering how it would all play out.

I just couldn't see how you'd get there, what steps you needed to take. It didn't seem easy or obvious in any way. There seemed to be too much for you to do.

Death, I felt, wasn't necessarily within your grasp.

July 9

I don't quite believe the philosopher Galen Strawson when he says: 'If, as an adult, I ask myself whether I'd rather be alive than dead tomorrow morning, and put aside the fact that some people would be unhappy if I were dead, I find, after reflection, in any normal, nondepressed period of life, that I have no preference either way.'

For Strawson, to be deprived of life – providing death is 'instant', 'painless', 'completely unexperienced', and 'completely unforeseen' – is to 'lose nothing'. It would make no difference if he were 'happy, or in love, or looking forward to something'. 'My future life and experience (the life and experience I will have if I don't die now),' he argues, 'don't belong to me in such a way that they're something that can be taken away from me.'

But if push came to shove, would he really have no preference either way? Even if one is unhappy, out of love, or has nothing to look forward to, there's a little something to be said for life, for nothing more than the experience of experience itself – the warmth of the sun on one's face, the smell of bread in the toaster.

And then there's you, of course, weeping in the garden, telling us all how you wish you'd had a chance to fight it.

July 10

Sense of:

   – do you realize what's happened? Do you know what you've done?

July 11

My first day back at work (phased return) sees me scuttling into the Department, heading straight for my office, shutting the door behind me, doing my little bit and then, when the voices in the corridor outside abate, stealing out the building and hurrying home, all without seeing or speaking to a single student or colleague.

July 12

Had, today, what could be described as a good day.

Started to worry about things again.

July 13

Attended an online grief support group this evening.

At the side of other people's (often multiple) losses, my own loss seemed paltry and insufficient, perfectly manageable. I worried that my grief wasn't good enough, that I'd no right to be there.

All the same, when the session came to an end, I didn't want to leave, found myself temporizing, typing 'thank you' and 'take care' into the chat box over and over, hoping the collective leave-taking would last forever …

I couldn't bring myself to click the red exit button – to return to my empty, silent room.

July 14

Those moments when I catch myself.

– He's dead.

July 15

Yes, you were big – 'Big Clive' – but there was more to you than your size and strength, even though you were happy to let these things define you. That muscular front belied a sharp mind and practical, philosophical wisdom. Unlike me, the arch sciolist, you weren't afraid to state that you didn't know what you didn't know. In fact, you made a point of it, cutting through my 'clever' arguments and reducing them to first principles with your Socratic questioning. Whenever I argued with you, I had to do away with my big words and trusty shibboleths, had to think on my own feet. I had the degree and the PhD and the articles in *Social Semiotics*, but yours was a fiercer intelligence, a deeper, more instinctive cleverness.

July 16

Mum and Dad try to carry on doing their usual things – the Friday night bar snack, the weekend trip into town.

When I phone them one late afternoon, Mum answers, mumbling through a mouthful of food.

I apologize for disturbing them.

'Don't worry, love', she says. 'You're not disturbing us. We're just having our prawn salads.'

Our prawn salads.

Never have I felt such love for my parents.

July 17

(Day at Sue and Graham's)

Note, from seeing the latest edition on the coffee table, that they still take the *Radio Times*.

(Succour in the tritest of continuities.)

July 18

I don't recall your last words. But somewhere towards the end I remember you telling me the new *Top Gun* film was out.

I went to see it a few weeks later. You didn't miss much. Wasn't much good. (Spoiler alert: Maverick saves the day.)

July 19

(Four months after)

I still hanker after some glimmering insight, still long to talk about him – with strangers especially (the man in the doorway, the woman at the park).

Someone, somewhere, holds the key.

July 21

Extract from Thomas Nagel's classic essay on death:

If we are to make sense of the view that to die is bad, it must be on the ground that life is a good and death is the corresponding deprivation or loss, bad not because of any positive features but because of the desirability of what it removes. We must now turn to the serious difficulties which this hypothesis raises … Essentially, there are three types of problem …

In many respects, I admire and feel I need this kind of writing, feel it's good for me. It is clear, rational, and precisely analytic ('there are three types of problem'). All the same, in my present state, there is something about it that irks me, or distracts me rather, something to do with its cool literalness and systematic abstraction, the way it treats death as though it were a counter in a game of logic. For I can't help inserting him – you – into the text, can't escape the emotive play of association and connotation that this impeccable kind of writing invariably seeks to suppress.

July 23
Tears throughout the morning and afternoon. Terrible day.

July 25
What is it to know that 'he is dead forever'?
   What does that fact demand of me?

July 29
In the weeks following the interment service, it feels as though he's drifting away, growing ever distant.
   I put this down not so much to anything like incipient closure as my increasing complacency with grief.

August 7
(Eight days in the Black Forest)

I thought that the thrill of departure (airport buzz and bustle, full English, a few pints before sunrise), followed by a spell in the land of fairy tales, might make up for things.

I was looking forward to walks in the deep dark woods, imagining myself retracing the footsteps of Little Snow White and Hansel and Gretel ...

But I soon discovered I was insusceptible to the charm of the place – my being there didn't square with his absence – and spent most of the week, to the annoyance of everyone else (*you just don't see us*), in a state of distracted torpor, wanting to get back to him, lost.

(Should've mugged up on my Grimm's. Not every trail of crumbs leads out of the dark forest.)

August 13

Tramping the otherwise lovely streets of Baden Baden, the far-flung unfamiliarity of the place ever reminding me that he is no longer here.

And then today, standing outside 46 Gernstrasse (an address of no historic or cultural significance, a place no more interesting than the more commercially oriented buildings surrounding it), I experience, if only for a moment, without end or object, without reason or design, something not unlike absolute joy and delight.

August 15

Sleepy taxi to the airport, silence reigning.

The same kind of silence when you and I took that early morning taxi to JFK twenty years ago. Too tired to talk, I spent the journey drooling slightly (the drooling, I remember the drooling), transfixed by the gold crucifix swinging from the rear-view mirror.

But, leaning over me from the back seat, you took an interest in him, you wanted to listen, to know his story – how he had left his family behind in Havana, hadn't seen them in a long time, but they needed the money and there were big dollars to be made in New York, and one day soon, sweet Jesus, he would seem them all again – of course he would see them! – these things were possible, everything was possible now.

August 16

Has the time come, to paraphrase Joan Didion, to let him go, to keep him dead?

What chance, otherwise, of beginning to live again?

August 17

His death remains unreal for me, an unconscionable affront. (And by rights, at two years older, I should have been the first to go.)

But if there had been any say in who gets to outlive the other, would I have put him first?

August 18

Spend, as I often do, part of the morning walking up and down the aisles of Poundland and B&M Bargains.

Somehow, among kitchen foil, shower curtains, and boxes of Toffifee, I can almost believe he isn't dead.

August 19

On the big screen in the overflowing sports bar, to the accompaniment of ecstatic whoops and cheers, someone scores a goal. And granted, it's a good goal, a great goal, right in the top corner!

But who here attaches any significance to the unavoidable fact that we all must die?

Too bad, isn't it?

August 20

(A walk in and around Kenton, South Devon)

It was dusk when we, just the dog and I, set off. By the time we picked up the trail out of the village, it was almost entirely dark, and I would've turned back if weren't for Frieda running on ahead, her amber eyes flashing back at me in the torchlight.

Presently, climbing through Powderham woods, we came across a clearing and then, standing desolately above the Exe Estuary, the old gothic folly. The tower had appeared solid and imposing in the distance, but now as I approached it, it seemed oddly insubstantial – like an elaborate piece of stage scenery which one firm push might send toppling over ... I knocked on the half-moonlit door (no answer) and shone my torch through a gap in the wall (nothing except wooden beams, straw on the ground – no phantom listeners, no you).

But as we walked round the rear of the structure, the dog stopped and barked at something moving in front of us ... a small figure ... a little ... a little ... a little girl ... a little girl, it seemed. Yes, a little girl. But it couldn't be a person, especially not a little girl, not here, not in the darkness, not a little girl ... As I drew closer – barely having time to ask myself what she was doing here and what I should do about it – I found myself looking into the sad, round eyes of Rapunzel, a painted wooden figure tied to the perimeter fence, shaking in the wind ... The dog came tentatively over, sniffed, seemed satisfied, and trotted on.

... Skirting the woods on the way back, stopped at an opening into the forest. Had no idea where it went, but wanted to go in – and go in deeply, unfathomably deep – to follow the trail wherever it led me, wherever he may be ... But by now it was getting late. I'd been out far longer than I said I would.

And yet the woods. The woods!

They were lovely, dark and lovely ...

I struck out for home.

They would be waiting for me.

August 21

The daily catechism.

> Say it.
> He's dead.

Good. Say it again.

He's dead.

Say it again.

He's dead.

Again.

He's dead.

Again.

Dead.

Again.

Dead.

Good. Good.

Now move on …

August 24

Up at 6 reading Hardy ('Poems of 1912–13', elegies for Emma). Rest of the house asleep. Mild tempest outside – dead leaves blowing about the yard.

The beguiling, bitter-sweet melancholy of the poems. Hardy's is a voice that, with its wistful repetitions and syntactical headiness, affords a strange comfort, comfort, nonetheless.

But I want more from Hardy. Want to confront loss on his terms, as he does, for him to do it for me.

Would that I might inhabit his yearning grief-scape as if it were my own!

September 13

Good news. New customers, I learn from the tanning store window display, are entitled to one free session on the sunbeds.

September 17

(Belgrade)

Just as I'm about to give my first ever plenary talk, he catches me off guard.

I look around the auditorium – not the largest of gatherings – and take in the audience, one by one:

You wouldn't have known him, of course. How could you? But the thing is, he's dead, my brother, or so they say. Sometimes he wrong foots me like this – he's good at that, my brother – was always, is always, messing around and playing childish pranks. (He once sneaked some dirty words into my undergraduate essay on T. S. Eliot, gave a whole new meaning to the objective correlative.)

No matter, no matter. He need not detain us, the bastard.

Then I begin.

September 18

Walking through Karađorđev Park after dinner.

Heard it (thumping baleful chanting) before I saw it (large shifting crowd in front of the Karađorđe Monument): the far-right demonstration which the conference delegates had warned me about.

Of course, I should've turned around, found another way back to my hotel. But I thought of you and all those extremist events you'd policed, and how you'd rib me for turning tail … So I carried on – your otherwise timid sibling, with his Richard Holloway under his arm, weaving his way through that fascist concourse, not really caring if it all kicked off, feeling in fact no so much relief when he safely came out the other side as disappointment – wanting to go back in again (again and again), utterly safe in the knowledge that, with you around, no one, but no one, would dare lay a finger on him.

September 25

Five months after his death, I still feel that I'm waiting for something to happen, for something to be clarified, for some huge significance to reveal itself.

September 29

All I can do is fold myself into, and huddle inside, the searingly sweet melancholy of it all (melancholy, melancholy – nothing wrong with melancholy). Doing so affords less comfort than protection, spares me the effort of suffering, of trying to work things through. (After all, what is mourning but work – the work, that is, 'of necessary failure'?)

October 7

Mum phones me early in the morning, shaken.

During the small hours she received a text message, purportedly from either you or me (and, of course, it wasn't me).

Hi mum, I'm texting you off a friend's phone. I've smashed mine and their phone's about to die, can you text my new number please …

Evidently, it's a scam – and a quick search online confirms so. She sounds disappointed when I tell her.

And yet on some level, I'm sure she still believes, as I do, that it could only have come from you.

October 10

I (still) don't hear him in the breeze or see him glinting on the snow.

I find him in the early episodes of *You've Been Framed* and the signature tune of *Mr Rossi* ('lala yala yala ya …').

October 13

Things I remember towards the end:

– Wondering whether your death was a good example of what the sociologist Philippe Ariès counter-intuitively called a 'wild death' – hidden, controlled, over-medicalized (opioids, syringe-driver, coma, and so on) – and if it were, whether we'd failed you.

– Overhearing the nurses in the cafeteria talking about things other than death and dying, and thinking: why shouldn't they talk about things other than death and dying? Why shouldn't they? Let them talk about Centre Parcs and musical theatre and Freddie's audition for *The Wizard of Oz*.

– The slow, deliberately slow (as if by going ever so slowly I might forever prolong it) walk back to your room.

– Stopping by the chapel, an unobtrusive and seemingly forgotten space that did its tender best (babbling brook sounds, interactive memory tree) to accommodate non-believers.

– The soft, welcoming carpet in reception – and how it soon (much too soon!) gave way to the hard linoleum of the inpatient wards: curt-symbolic transition from life to death.

– Your name on the door, among all the other names on the doors – the Maureens, Mavises, and Normans: the names of a generation slightly more suited to death.

– Thinking at the moment of your death that this was the most exhilarating thing that had ever happened to me, that everything in my life had been leading up to something like this, and that though brothers die all the time, I should be singularly honouring your death, taking it all down, noting for example the way the sunlight came in through the open blinds and the unaccustomed orange stubble on your face, because otherwise I might forget these things, and you wouldn't want me to forget these things – though come to think of it, knowing you, you'd be quite happy if I did forget them, especially the stubble.

– Staring at the clock on the wall for a while – five twenty-five, it said – as if taking in the time of death might somehow prove vital in the future.

– The stillness in the room.

– Realizing winter had passed.

– Not knowing what to do.

What does one do?

October 26

Six months after his mother's death, Barthes records in his diary that his suffering is still chronically acute – hardened into an enduring sadness and painful acedia.

What do I feel at this six-month juncture? Whereas Barthes, for all his acedia, maintained his searing perception, I feel I've reached a point (some sort of culmination?) where I'm largely unable to think for myself, must rely on the thoughts of others – whatever it is that needs to be thought about, pondered, considered, assessed …

November 5

Let us play a little language game. Let us see if we can bring you back.

Bertrand Russell (who loved parsing silly sentences) said that the statement 'The king of France is bald' is false. It is false, he reasoned, for there is no present king of France (France, of course, has long been a republic).

By the same token, 'My brother is dead' must be false, for there is no present brother.

And so, if the sentence 'My brother is dead' is false, it follows that you cannot be dead …

… No, it doesn't work.

Because: if there is no present brother, then 'My brother is not dead' must also be false (a statement and its negation, you see, I think, cannot both be false).

So what's the answer? Are you alive or are you dead? (I lose track of these things.)

Well, according to Bertie, you should be dead. For you cannot be treated as a referring expression in disguise. You can only take the form of a grammatical subject. Nothing more, I'm afraid.

All the same, if Russell's logical form can't save you, I'll gladly settle for a grammatical formula that keeps you alive, that continues to premise your existence.

You are … He is …

Either will do.

November 9

One of the reasons why grief shakes us so much, writes philosopher Michael Cholbi, is because 'we tend to build our practical identities around the existence of other people, those whose existences are contingent, but then forget that fact'.

I think of our lives running alongside each other, our parallel lives, close, but often apart, never converging enough.

I in my corner feeding, working, sleeping … You in yours …

The routineness of it all, the taken-for-grantedness (because I never noticed, because I was 'looking away!').

To have known then what I know now.

November 15

Like Hardy, I'm drawn to old haunts.

Three months after the death of his first wife, Emma Gifford, Hardy made a pilgrimage to Cornwall, revisiting and writing about the scenes of their courtship – places such as Boscastle ('At Castle Boterel') and St Juliot ('St Launce's Revisited'). Inspired by his pilgrimage – and the nostalgic yearning of these Cornish poems – I find myself returning to our old haunts, to the Frankie and Benny's and Nando's off Redfield Way, and the adjoining Showcase Cinema, all of them unremarkable places in themselves, but places possessed of a 'strange necromancy', places where we spent so much time together.

Revisiting these old haunts, I thought I'd feel your loss more acutely (hence more exquisitely). But now that I'm here, tucked away in our favourite booth at F&B's, with my Collected Hardy and pint of Peroni, your absence feels no more acute than it does in other places. What I feel I suppose is a kind of vague melancholy, a blank but not unpleasant sadness. (I try to conjure you here, sitting across from me, your thick thigh, as it used to, bulging out from the under the table, the waiters having to sidestep it.)

No doubt you'd think my nostalgic obsession with the past unhealthy, a form of avoidance, a way of sparing myself the heavy work of moving on. But there's an adaptive dimension to nostalgia – psychologists tell us that its therapeutic potential is often overlooked. Living in the past, they argue, is not a 'feeble retreat' or an 'escape from reality' but a resource, a 'coping mechanism for the bereaved'. Engaging in nostalgic reverie, so the argument goes, is an act of narrative meaning making that 'nurtures social connectedness' and enhances self-assurance, which in turn 'raises optimism …'

So, for the time being, you'll find me in one of our favourite places, doing my sentimental best 'to re-establish psychological homeostasis in the aftermath of distress'.

November 21

Rain.

All through November it has rained – willed, adamant, implacable rain.

It will be raining now on his small, overcrowded plot, on the plants and flowers, the pinwheels and electric candles, the Brussels sprouts and packs of protein powder, the painted stones and little dogs, the photographs and tins of Red Bull, and the cellophane-wrapped birthday card ('To a Special Son. 49 Today!').

(Paul Stanbridge: 'Is it perhaps easier to die than ever to tend to the dead?')

December 2

Late evening (with few people about).

Loiter for a little while outside the tanning store, trying to summon the critical will to semiotically unpack the window display … with its heady preponderance of warm colours (naturally!), gently rounded, friendly informal fonts, and close-ups of tanned, happy participants, all of whom look amiably at the viewer, a visual address that speaks symbolically, though illusorily, of affinity and affiliation. *You too can have/can be …*

(Such seductive play and exchange of 'embodied sign-values'!)

Despair.

Absolute despair.

December 5

Christmas looms.

Around early December, we would text each other lines from *The Box of Delights* – an exchange he would always initiate, ever keen at this time of year to summon the brumal world of Chester Hills and Bottlers Down.

> The wolves are running …
> I say, that's the purple pim!

This year we don't let anything as paltry as death spoil our silly little ritual: I simply text him the first quotation, commence proceedings on his behalf.

> Time and tide and buttered eggs wait for no man …

December 7

Turning to my body more and more.

The habit I've developed (when alone) of pressing down on my lower premolars as hard as I can.

They never move.

Their sheer solidity, their utter rootedness and dependability.

December 11

The death business notwithstanding, I grew to like the hospice.

Wandering about its mazy, neon-lit corridors, Schubert's Piano Trio No. 2 looping in my head, I felt as if I were in a Kubrick movie, felt lost yet acutely half alive. In the long echoey spaces, I began to appreciate the regularity of my footfall and the wholesome length of my stride, the steady efficiency with which I could cover ground (no one would have covered ground here like

I was covering it now) … The more I explored the building, the more I felt I might reveal some hidden ontological truth about it, certify the place, make it real (or more real) for us both.

(You, no doubt, 'Oh fuck off with your Schubert and your Kubrick and your existential crap.')

December 16

I should know – because I was there. That last breath of yours (prolonged, testy, overstatedly yawny) was not so much confirmation as performance.

At any rate (and this is the point, I think), it did nothing to firm my belief in the absoluteness of your death.

December 18

Going back over these notes, am struck by the recurring use of the second person.

A perfectly natural choice of pronoun, of course, but who exactly am I talking to when I address no-longer 'you'?

December 20

Walking down the street this morning, I shouted 'fuck' out loud.

It's not like me. It's not like me at all.

I put it down to the constant weather.

That, and to what Elisabeth Kübler-Ross calls the death-adjustment pattern. (It's not uncommon, EK-R suggests, to be angry during the grief cycle, to unload your rage on the environment – yes, it's all a vital part of the healing process, a positive sign that you're accepting the reality of your loss.)

Hence: I am accepting my loss.

December 24

Midnight.

Picture, once again, those six mystifying sprouts that turned up in my rogan josh.

Was it you? Could it really have been you?

Still hoping it might be so.

December 31

'The year is going, let him go …'

2023

January 1

You're dead, you old bastard.

How come? How hard is it to stay alive, to keep on going? Most of us manage it. It's something we tend to do every day, and you'd been doing it well enough for forty-eight years.

Now look at you!

Yes, yes, the sympathy cards spoke of your 'brave fight' and your 'battling hard' and things like that. But, by extension, you didn't fight hard enough. For you lost the battle! Granted, it was a battle you had little chance of winning. But couldn't you have fought harder? After all, far lesser mortals have beaten cancer.

I doubt whether the well-wishers were aware of the implications of their choice of trope, a metaphor that sees medicine as war and illness as a battle. But its recurring use demonstrates just how entrenched this pernicious figure of speech has become in everyday discourse. I've never liked it, and have grown to dislike it even more after you were taken ill. It plagued us all the way.

The doctors spoke of hitting you with the strongest drugs they had, of throwing everything at you. You were big enough to take it, and, of course, you'd take anything! To do otherwise would have been to give up the fight, to concede defeat. And besides, those twin treatments – nivolumab and ipilimumab – sounded so potent, so proficient, so clinically alluring. ('It's costing them over a hundred grand!' you said after your first infusion, astonished that such an amount was being spent on you.)

But like I did – though my fatigue was purely linguistic – you soon grew battle weary. The endless batteries of tests and biopsies, the arsenals of drugs and therapies …

Perhaps this punishing regimen gave you a little more time, a few extra weeks, but it tore you apart, ultimately proved fruitless.

And yet even after it had failed, the pressure to carry on pursuing some form of 'medical doing something' never abated. I recall the well-intentioned doctor calling you one evening and asking, in tentatively carneying tones, if you could 'just' get yourself down to A&E. They would do something for you, he insisted, scan your back again, give you more radiotherapy.

You were lying supine on the sofa, unimprovably comfy, but unable to move, a fact you fruitlessly relayed over and over. 'Mate,' you said, rolling your eyes in despair, 'I'm going nowhere.'

'But if you could just …'

A week later, you were dead.

It was a gentle death.

A good death.

It was your victory.

January 8

More idealized models in the tanning store window this morning.

Stop and delight (once again) in the allure of embodied sign-values, the subtle interplay of seduction and self-expression, and, beneath it all, the understated but irresistible injunction to see oneself in terms of 'an ideal future tanned "You"'.

Happy Tanuary, C!

January 15

Walking the dog (late at night in the park).

If there's no one around, I run towards the trees in the distance.

Perhaps if I reach them in time (I say to myself), I might catch him there.

No luck so far. He always seems to elude me …

Still, I don't give up on surprising him sometime.

And so, once again, as I did this evening, I find myself running from tree to tree in the darkness, the dog (half-elated, half-afraid) barking after me.

January 16

Learn belatedly of the death of Victor Lewis Smith, the anarchic, boundary-pushing satirist and broadcaster. I always delighted in his chutzpah – the utterly fearless way in which he ridiculed the pompous and powerful.

The obituaries in the press spoke of his having 'a short illness' – a circumlocution that didn't seem to square with his fierce temerity and impertinence, a phrase to me synonymous with the disease that dare not mention its name.

No such pussy footing around your death! Everyone knew what it was. Cancer! Cancer! Cancer, folks! – Cancer all the way! All the way!

But though it did for thee, cancer (the noun, the name) held absolutely no power over you. As a linguist, I admired the free and easy and open way you used it – in your hands it was a mere signifier, a bloodless referent, a token, a word disarmed of its sting. Only by talking openly about cancer, I recall once saying to you (rather donnishly), will we increase our understanding of the disease, demystify and lessen the stigma surrounding it.

All the same, I couldn't help recoil when I read about your illness in the village newsletter:

'… cancer which had taken control over his body.'

January 18

Walking past Wetherspoons on my way to work, catch sight of several figures sitting alone with their pints, all staring forlornly into the distance. What anguish, I wonder, sustains them?

Contemplate taking the morning off, abandoning work on my Chomsky lecture, and taking my place among them (after all, even though it's been almost a year now, surely I'm still entitled to start early?).

But I push on.

Such is the pull of transformational grammar.

January 21

Second dream about him – absurd dream in which I find myself on the set, a giant water tank, of the 1992 film *Under Siege* (a movie neither of us cared for).

I'm being shown around by burly leading actor Steven Seagal, who seems to be in awe of and eager to impress me (something no doubt to do with you, with you being my brother). The two of us, Seagal and I, are travelling around the set in a small yellow dinghy, and Seagal is concerned that the machine-generated waves are going to tip us over at any moment. But during calmer intervals, when he's not holding on so tightly, he insists on showing me the size of his biceps – which, admittedly, are big – and he talks about you constantly. He wants to pass on his bodybuilding advice, does Seagal – tips, he thinks, you'll find 'extremely significant'.

And yet listen encouragingly to Seagal as I do, I haven't the heart to tell him that you're dead, that, as much as he insists I do, I cannot pass on his advice.

January 24

Cancer could never kill you. No, not you!

Weren't you always telling me that you were invincible, that there was a side-stepping immortality about you, an untouchable, inviolable strength?

Oh, how it blundered! In you, it was up against the impossible!

What chance did it have against you – you of the super-human qualities!

January 27

Reading W. S. Graham. Am particularly taken by 'Dear Bryan Wynter':

This is only a note
To say how sorry I am
You died. You will realize
What a position it puts

Me in. I couldn't really
Have died for you if so
I were inclined. The carn
Foxglove here on the wall
Outside your first house
Leans with me standing
In the Zennor wind.

Anyhow how are things?
Are you still somewhere
With your long legs
And twitching smile under
Your blue hat walking
Across a place? Or am
I greedy to make you up
Again out of memory?
Are you there at all?
I would like to think
You were all right
And not worried about
Monica and the children
And not unhappy or bored.

It's all too easy to substitute you, CH, for BW, and fling the same kind of questions at you.

But Graham's poem is more than a heuristic for addressing the dead. It's a testament, CH, to the compensatory power of everyday language, the succour of mundanity.

All those phatic phrases – see how they maintain the one-sided dialogue for people like me (for you dead don't seem to reply), how they keep things together when loneliness and longing threaten to overwhelm.

This is what phatic talk does, CH. It's not aimless chatter. The words of the shambling figure in the park have direction – he directs them against the silence.

His words are a 'mode of action', a 'bond of union' (as the great Malinowski put it).

They are all he has.

January 29

Robert D. Richardson's *Three Roads Back: How Emerson, Thoreau, and William James responded to the Greatest Losses of Their Lives*.

– Henry David Thoreau's brother, John, died from tetanus at the age of twenty-seven.

– In the aftermath, Thoreau took to his bed for four weeks, but thereafter rallied quickly, buoyed by his devotion to the natural world, his consoling love of woods, fields, ponds, and the like.

– 'What had been a more or less conventional romantic approach to nature,' Richardson writes, 'quickly became, after John's death, a profoundly felt emotional acceptance – not just an intellectual assent – of death as an inescapable part of living, and an acceptance that at some level, there is no death. The very process of decay is a life process … This conviction, once firmly accepted, is, paradoxically, a powerful force for individual resilience.'

– Perhaps if I embrace Thoreau's divinity of nature, his 'force for individual resilience', I, too, can shorten the span of recovery, confine it, as he did, to little more than six months.

Whatever the case, HD, I promise I'll try to love nature more often.

January 31

Is cancer, as the surgeon and writer Sherwin Nulan claims, 'amoral' and 'immoral'? Is it 'evil'?

Much as I understand the need to render cancer in such visceral terms, to personify it, simplify it, we should be wary of readily assigning malign agency to the disease – cancer as 'criminal', 'killer', 'demon', 'terrorist', 'predator', and so on.

My brother was neither possessed by a demon nor the victim of crime. Those cancerous cells in his body were not witting miscreants – wily intruders intent on outsmarting his immune system. They were his own cells growing (as cells do) inside him.

(Fergus Shanahan: 'Ascribing a cunning deviousness to cancer frightens patients and is biologically meaningless.')

All the same – fuck you, cancer. Fuck you.

February 3

To Twickenham to join old friends who'd invited me to watch the rugby.

Not caring if I was late (have little interest in sporting events, nor did I relish the prospect of a long evening devoted to reminiscing about you and the good old days), I deliberately missed the train. Deliberately missed the next train, too. And the one after that, spending the intervening hour or so reading Paul Stanbridge's *My Mind To Me A Kingdom Is* on the platform ... When the fourth train pulled into the station, I finally felt duty bound to board it. (Strong desire, all the same, to miss every London-bound train in perpetuity.)

On the tube heading towards East Hounslow, I became aware of a voice speaking somewhere to the side of me. It was evidently close by – for I could make out each word distinctly – but no matter how many times I surveyed the space around me, I couldn't pinpoint the mouth from which the words were emanating. There were several candidates – mouths whose movements were roughly in sync with the words I was hearing – mouths, moreover, that seemed to be speaking in concert, speaking the same or similar words – words at least of the same articulatory shape and appearance. (Was this your doing? Some sort of diablerie on your part?) For the remainder of the journey, I had to close my eyes and put my hands over my ears …

At Hounslow I took a couple of drinks. (You wouldn't have begrudged me a few analeptic swigs.) But time flies when you're reeling from unannounced psychogenic shock, and I didn't feel like rushing my recovery. A few drinks became four, became five … and a few more after that.

… By the time I got to Twickenham, thoroughly in my cups, the rugby had finished (that was one thing at least). Crowds were spilling out of the stadium and on to the streets. Rather than seek out our old friends directly – they were waiting for me at the Toyota garage across the way – I stepped into the throng and, not caring where it took me, let myself be carried away.

March 2

Even in illness you excelled. There was something about your cancer – it always seemed clean to me, immaculate. I never thought of it in terms of corruption or mutation, a dirty violation. There was always something natural, virtuous – a certain nobility about it.

March 3

It's around this time of year that sprouts go out of season.

March 5

Stopping by the tanning store this evening, I note that if one makes a block booking (supposedly a good thing to do), one is entitled to 50 per cent extra tanning time.

March 7

'a certain nobility about it' – nonsense, of course. But for both our sakes (mine especially), I have to try to explain away your rotten disease.

March 25

(Weekend at Mum and Dad's)

Desperate for a shave, and having forgotten to bring my razor with me, I went through the cupboards in the bathroom – and came across your old shaving gear: foams, gels, blades, after shaves, all of which must have been over thirty years old. ('The people leave and the things stay'.)

I tried one of the capless, rusty tins. It hissed a little, ever so faintly at first, but as I continued to press down on the nozzle, my hand on your hand, the old thing wheezed and coughed into life again, emitting a small burst of liquid foam – not enough for one of your 'legendary' close shaves, but enough at least to rid me of my infernal itch.

April 11

My brother and I are having a bite in Nando's.

He asks me if I remember the fight.

Yes, I say, putting down my Hardy, I remember the fight. How could I forget the fight? The lads piling in over there, tables and chairs everywhere, diners fleeing (like a brawl in a Western saloon, we said afterwards). I remember you getting up from the table, reluctantly leaving your buttered chicken, and your dead feet walking into the melee, with me trailing at a distance, thinking we'd both be done over, for it was that kind of a melee – look, see, here's one with a chair above his head, raising it higher and higher (spoilsport you: removing it from him just when he's fully cocked) – and here's one with a blade, and another (I knew there'd be knives) – and now I've lost you – where are you? – you're in deep, thick and tight among them, sorting things out from the centre – but all I can see is a pack of baseball caps, the young in one another's arms, you in there somewhere … And now, as I feared, there's blood … there's blood on the floor – plenty of blood – is it yours? – I remember thinking it was yours, certain it was yours (you've so much more of it to lose), and hence assuming here ends our evening out, the meal, the cinema, the pick 'n' mix … But, no, it isn't your blood, for they're peeling away from you now, sprinting for the door – and lo! look! – there you are, seemingly unscathed, checking yourself over, dusting yourself down – and yes, God knows how, you *are* unscathed …

When you finally return to your chicken, the youths having fled, the police since arrived, 'It's still warm', you say, chuckling to yourself, resuming where you left off.

April 21

(The anniversary)

I think of the all things you've missed this year: the new steakhouse on Queen Street, Forest in the Premiership, meals at Amores, Mum's Sunday roasts, winter sunrises over Oakham, *John Wick: Chapter 4.*

But as the great Emil Cioran once observed, we shouldn't pity you, you dead, for your lot have cracked every problem, starting, of course, 'with the problem of death.'

May 27

These notes are becoming more and more scarce – in Barthes's phrase, 'silting up'.

Evidence perhaps not so much of increasing closure, as of their having passed their grieve-by date?

June 3

I used to worry about you, your routines.

All that creatine and protein powder, all those energy drinks and chemical-laden supplements, all those impossible weights (at your age!).

But when I questioned you about these things, you reassured me, my brother. Told me not to worry.

Told me you were a machine.

August 5

Still think of him constantly, but all the same I feel a distance (not solely temporal) opening up between us – sense of his breaking away, growing detached, of my being able to go on without him.

As Barthes (fifteen months after his mother's death) put it: 'We don't forget, but something *vacant* settles in us.'

August 6

Leave off, he tells me. Let me be.

We dead are happy to be alone.

September 22

That morning when I slipped into your house, called out your name and, hearing no reply, went upstairs to find you fitfully sleeping in the spare room, the windows tightly shut, the death-white curtains drawn. Rather than wake you, I watched you for a while, watched you in your restless sleep, and I remember thinking, you lucky basket, you'll soon be shot of all this, but I'll have to go on, I'll have to go on living, living and partly living. Never mind your twitching and wheezing, it's muggins here who'll have to see to things, me who'll have to shoulder the burden – the house, Mum and Dad, and whatever else is (inevitably) coming down the track …

… Downstairs, I pored over your long list of medications.

Perhaps one of them would save us.

December 1

Seeing a child's basketball hoop – little index of familial love – on a driveway stops me short.

Where have I been all these months?

December 11

Approaching death, how does one meaningfully live out whatever time remains?

Moments before he drank the hemlock that killed him, Socrates was learning to play a new melody on the flute.

'What's the point in that?' somebody asked him.

'To know this song before dying', he replied.

One of your last text messages instructed me to: 'bring Arnie book'. 'Arnie book' was Arnold Schwarzenegger's *Encyclopedia of Modern Bodybuilding*. For a while, you'd been thinking about making a series of weight training podcasts, and were now beginning to sketch out content for them. You'd never podcasted before, didn't really know what you were doing, but were determined, as you put it, in mock-Wildean terms, to declare your genius to the universe ...

And there were the birthday meals, the cinema trips, the (still) super-heavy weightlifting, the weekend getaways, the endless Amazon parcels (what did you do with it all?) and the holiday in Turkey, which never came about but, in your eyes at least, remained an ever-present prospect.

You always had your plans, your projects. Your never-ending plans and projects.

To know this song before dying.

December 16

'Tis the season to be tanned' proclaims the poster in the tanning store window.

December 23

Is forty-eight years really a good age to die?

'It's not much of an age', somebody said to me at the wake.

'Maybe', I might've replied, 'but it's a little better than forty-five. Better still than forty-two and forty. And as sure as you and I are combing the length and breadth of this buffet (yes – yes, he'd have been first in the queue), it beats thirty-five, thirty-three, thirty-one, and thirty, to say nothing of twenty-nine, twenty-five, twenty-one, eighteen, seventeen, and sixteen, which are all paltry by comparison. And anything under ten, well, that's slight by anybody's standards.'

'Crude quantitative judgements apart,' I might've continued, 'nothing can undo the fact that he lived, that (to quote the great W. N. P. Barbellion, who was a mere thirty when he died) he "telescoped" into his 48 years a "tolerably long life": he loved and was loved; he wept and enjoyed, struggled and overcame, and when the time came, he was not afraid, was even content, to die.'

'"Darest thou now O soul, Walk out with me toward the unknown region, Where neither ground is for the feet nor any path to follow?"

– Whitman, by the way.'

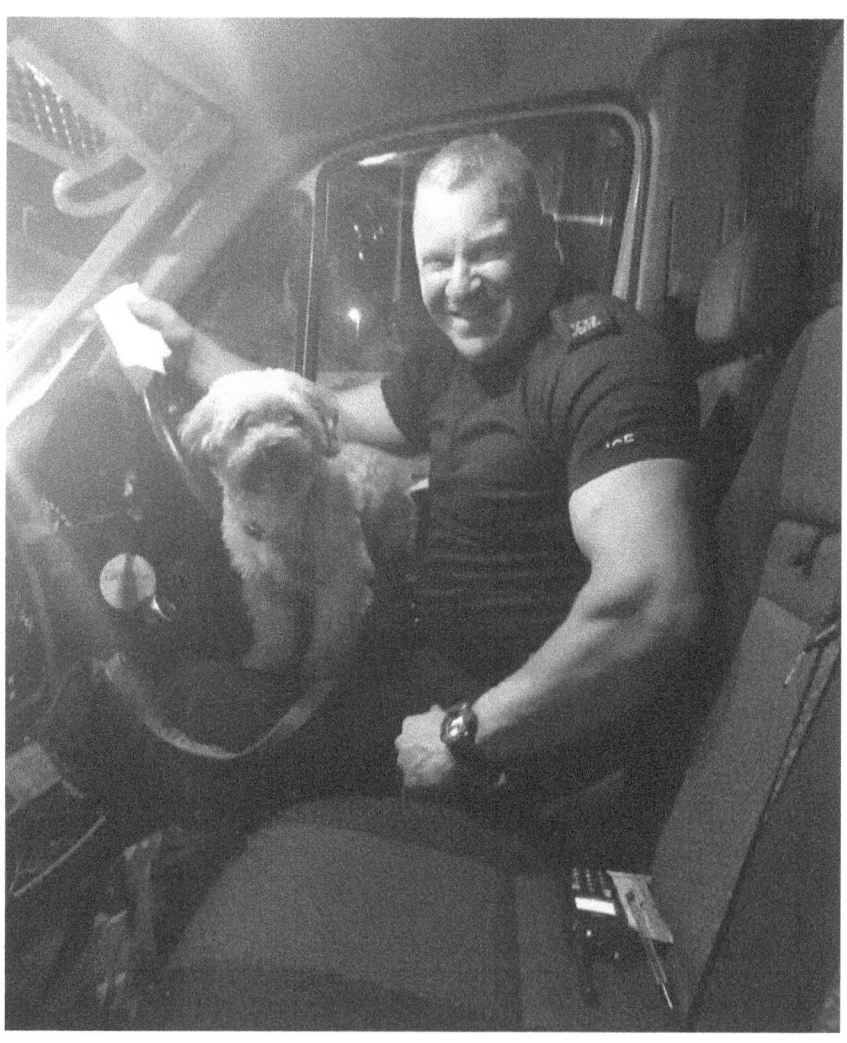

In lieu of a conclusion:
Four short postscripts

1

Jane Davis retired from The Reader in December 2022 after heading the organization for twenty-five years. She now devotes her time to gardening at Liverpool's beautiful Calderstones Park (the home of The Reader), where she keeps in touch with old colleagues and volunteers. 'We don't talk about shared reading', she said when I caught up with her recently online. 'We talk about roses. But if it's very bad weather, we'll read a poem.'

She continues, too, to lead a weekly online reading group that she's been running since lockdown. 'I absolutely adore it. We read Wordsworth's *The Prelude* over two years and we're now reading *Paradise Lost*.'

When I first interviewed Davis back in 2015, there was one question I forgot to ask her (in fact there were several questions I forgot to ask her). What did she make, I'd wanted to know, of the criticism often levelled at bibliotherapy that it treats mental health problems as merely individual concerns? During our Zoom call some nine years later, I finally put it to her that bibliotherapy initiatives such as shared reading are liable to overlook the environmental factors that give rise to mental illness and distress in the first place.

'I think that's true,' she told me. 'I think that the things that make us ill or unhappy often are poverty: poverty of expectation, poverty of education, poverty of self-understanding, economic poverty – all of those things are connected – and not only connected with poor people: I've met that in some very, very wealthy people as well. I'm not saying we can fix it, but what we're saying is that it [shared reading] might give you a language.' (By 'language' Davis means not language per se – but specifically language used 'to describe complex experience', the language of 'deeper, wider, and richer' thinking that, she argues, 'literature offers'.)

'I just think giving people access to language who don't have it is quite a revolutionary thing', she went on. 'Now whether you can then prove people use it or do something with it, I have no idea. And I do know that I've seen many people over many years not getting better or their situations get worse … So you might well say, "Shared reading did nothing!"'

She paused, then added, 'But I don't believe that, because the actual experience, whatever the rest of everything else is, is of value. I believe that because people I've been in groups with have told me that.'

Towards the end of our catch-up, I asked Davis whether she'd got everything out of shared reading that she'd wanted to get out of it.

'I would've been really chuffed if we'd managed to make it a statutory requirement that people in care homes and children's homes read to their residents', she replied, a little ruefully. 'But we're about two hundred years away from that. It's not even on the horizon.'

'But I do feel really glad and grateful that I got great literature out of the university – and for all the times when some wonderful poem had been read somewhere where that would never have happened.'

2

Angel Row Library permanently closed in 2020. Its closure passed me by, but I was able to visit the place one last time when, for a few days in April 2022, it hosted a sale of its old stock (mainly CDs, DVDs, and magazines). Devoid of books and patrons, the library was unrecognizable – it was hard to imagine that this was once the place where I swam 'from lure to lure' and the air 'seemed golden with the fellowship and grateful presence of other people'. There were no ghosts, no real memories, no matter how hard I tried to conjure them. I stayed for no more than twenty minutes, picking up on my way out, for fifty pence, a CD of Beethoven's Overtures (which like all my other untouched classical CDs, I knew I'd never listen to).

The sale wouldn't make much money. But Nottingham City Council needed to raise funds any which way it could. The Council's financial difficulties had continued to increase over the years, such that, in November 2023, it was forced to declare itself bankrupt (a situation the Tory government blamed on Council mismanagement, but which the Council blamed on shortfalls in government funding). Still, despite its parlous financial situation, the Council was able to invest in a new £10 million central library, which opened on 28 November 2023, the day before the local authority filed for bankruptcy.

Since the Covid pandemic, many libraries have reported lower user numbers. When I visited the new Central Library for the first time this summer, there was no sign that users were failing to return. The new glass-and-steel building was all civic purr, each of its three floors busily occupied by people at open desks and computer terminals, in reading rooms and study spaces – people of different ages and ethnicities, families, children, refugees. 'Yes, it's busier than the old place', one of the librarians told me as I nosed around. 'We've had about a thousand people a day since we opened', before adding: 'And the place doesn't leak.'

The library is undeniable impressive. It's bright, full of silver light, spacious and open, but also replete with secret spaces (spaces in which I could imagine a disillusioned bobby plotting their escape from the police service). 'There's so much more going off here', the librarian continued. 'There's an immersive room, where you can talk to Lord Byron, a concert space, a storytelling room, conference rooms, cafes, kids' playground, and miles and miles of bookshelves.'

I'll say it again: the library is impressive.

But as I write this (August 2024), I learn that the local authority is planning further library cuts, a move aimed at generating £1.5 million worth of savings over the next few years. Time will tell what material impact the cuts will have on people's lives. For now, at least, the new library continues to be a flagship of civic renewal in an otherwise run-down part of the city, a beacon that reaches a more varied audience than any other cultural platform on the high street.

3

What became of Robert?

According to his daughters, he's doing well. I visited him last summer at his new home in the south of England. I wasn't sure if he knew who I was (he doesn't always recognize Rachel and Susan), but he nonetheless seemed pleased to see me, was his old playful, amiable self. ('You've got a good one there!' he said, nodding towards my newly shaven head.)

When the moment came, I took out my yellow folder of poems and began to read Wordsworth's 'Daffodils' aloud, hoping that the poem would take him as it had taken him before. But this time my reading of the text seemed to leave him cold, to pass over him – at any rate, he was soon up and off, off out the dining room and down along the wide corridor that circles the perimeter of the care home. Instinctively, I went after him, still reading 'The Daffodils' aloud in his wake – I had to know whether he was still receptive to metered poetry – but now he was gliding towards the siren sound of music ahead of us … a seventies disco, as it happened, into which, despite my efforts to entice him back, he wandered with happy abandon … And that was the last I saw of him (dancing: dancing to the irresistible rhythms of Gloria Gaynor and the Bee Gees).

It was clear to me that Robert and his fellow residents were treated with great dignity and affection. The home is a model of person-centred care. Robert is also fortunate to have children who advocate on his behalf and who visit him regularly. But apart from his two daughters, he receives few other visitors. Many of his friends and acquaintances have severed contact with him completely: they see no point in maintaining contact with someone who no longer knows who they are. (They're not alone. According to a recent Alzheimer's Society survey, over 40 per cent of people believe it's pointless visiting friends and relatives with advanced dementia.)

It's curious. I suspect that his friends' staying away has as much to do with their anxieties about dementia as it does with the 'strain' of spending time with him. Whatever the case, I can understand their reluctance to visit Robert, and I don't judge them. There is a rational argument for not visiting a friend or relative in the advanced stages of cognitive decline. If the person no longer recognizes you, how can they be in a relationship with you? 'Heartless as it may seem,' writes philosopher Claudia Mills, 'I see little point in spending extensive time with someone who does not know me for who I am. To do so is to engage in a pretence that a relationship still continues that, tragically, is gone forever.'

But why is it pointless to continue such a relationship? For whom is it pointless? To visit and spend time with someone is 'proof that we exist for other people'. And besides, there is abundant evidence that people with advanced dementia benefit from receiving visits from friends and family. Visits induce feelings of well-being, feelings that endure for some time afterwards, 'even when the memory of the visit has been lost'. The need for social contact, moreover, is greater for people living with dementia than it is for most other individuals: the former are more liable to experience chronic loneliness. Dementia imposes barriers to maintaining existing relationships and forging new ones.

Spending time with Robert is never a chore. He might not recognize me 'in a narrowly cognitive sense', to quote dementia scholar Janelle Taylor, but he does recognize me as someone who is present with him, 'someone familiar perhaps'. And though his language has become increasingly abstruse, shorn of shared reference, there is still a knowingness to his words – his talk has a clear significance for him. The interaction's the thing, whatever the content.

And then there's gratitude. I don't, of course, have any filial obligation to visit Robert. But all the same I owe him a debt of gratitude, am grateful for the time we spent together and for what he taught me. Robert showed me how to read poetry aloud, encouraged me to meet a poem on its own terms, made me, in short, a better, more generous reader.

4

I believe now that my brother is dead. The passing days (852 to be precise) would seem to confirm it. At any rate, he has yet to return. But I love him still and know he still loves me.

Since his death I've done a lot of walking. Not walking in the rambling, coast-to-coast, three peaks challenge sense, but mundane, everyday walking – through and around the town centre and local housing estates, in parks and shopping centres and department stores, and up and down, over and over, the long silent corridors of the university. The thing to do, I've realized, has been to move constantly from place to place, the simple act of upping and going doing me good. Like it does for the grieving characters in David Grossman's *Falling Out of Time*, walking hints at the impossible possibility of seeing the dead again, perhaps even talking with them (who knows?), each sortie, in its own way, 'a journey of memorialization'.

Like many works of imaginative literature I've read in the wake of my brother's death, *Falling Out of Time* showed me that, in the face of loss, we cannot grow, cannot live without grief. Not to suffer grief is to be deprived of an experience that, although agonizing, is in some way good and peculiarly human. ('If one had a pill that would "wipe out" the grief of a bereaved friend,' writes Michael Cholbi, 'it would seem wrong to offer it to the friend.' To grieve is to be afforded a privileged 'route to our pasts. In grief's absence, we risk being irreversibly alienated from our personal histories.')

One cannot read oneself out of grief, of course. All the same, reading gave me direction, offered possible scripts and schemas. For it's not easy to talk to the dead. (What does one say?) Reading was a way of seeing things I wouldn't otherwise have seen, a way of picturing you, addressing you, summoning you more clearly, more thoroughly (locating you, that is, in places, those hidden recesses, where I would never have thought to look for you).

The unusually eloquent accounts of others, so much more than any theoretical model of mourning (grief doesn't always progress in certain discrete stages) seemed to validate my own experience. Reading helped me to understand what was happening to me, helped transform my often vague and inexpressibly private anguish into a more cogent narrative. Reading, to paraphrase Fernando Pessoa, offered relief from life, without actually relieving me of the business of living.

Yes, I worried that all this reading was spoiling things, was getting in between you and me, and that consequently I wasn't approaching you as you, you on your own terms. I worried that all I was doing was refracting and seeing you through the prism of literature, reducing everything to anecdotes and aperçus, to text and quotations, a never-ending set of references.

All that reading! At times, it felt as if other people's losses were more real to me than my own. (But therein, I suppose, C, lies one of the solaces of literature.)

The time of the dead is supposedly different from ours. You dead, C, are said to have fallen out of time, to live outside time, while my time stubbornly continues. What do we do, you and I, with these two temporalities? How do we reconcile them?

At the end of *Time Lived, Without Its Flow*, Denise Riley describes how her time and the time of her dead son are not two distinct temporalities but one: 'the time of the dead is, from now on, freshly contained within your own'.

No neat solution, no quick and easy remedy, of course. But it's a quite beautiful notion, a wonderful formation for holding the living and the dead together.

To know your time has become my own.

READING AND DEMENTIA:
POEMS FOR READING ALOUD

Below is a list of poems, freely available on the internet, that I have read in dementia care settings over the years. All are a joy to read aloud and all, in their own way, have connected with audiences. Once learned by heart at school, many of the poems will be well known to older generations – poetry, as Catherine Robson puts it, that beats as one with the body 'in measured familiarity'. But poetry, of course, doesn't have to be familiar for it to be appreciated and enjoyed. Hence the appearance of lesser-known and more contemporary poems, poems no less memorable, no less quotable, than their classic counterparts.

A. A. Milne, 'Halfway Down'

Adrian Mitchell, 'Stufferation'

A. E. Housman, 'Loveliest of Trees'

Alfred Lord Tennyson, 'The Charge of the Light Brigade'

Alfred Lord Tennyson, 'Crossing the Bar'

Alfred Lord Tennyson, 'The Eagle'

Alfred Lord Tennyson, 'Ulysses'

Benjamin Zephaniah, 'Talking Turkeys'

Charles Causley, 'Timothy Winters'

Charles Wolfe, 'The Burial of Sir John Moore after Corunna'

Christina Rossetti, 'Remember'

Claude McKay, 'December, 1919'

Edgar Allan Poe, 'Annabel Lee'

Edgar Allan Poe, 'The Raven'

Edward Lear, 'The Jumblies'

Edward Lear, 'The Owl and the Pussy-Cat'

E. E. Cummings, 'Maggie and Milly and Molly and May'

Elizabeth Barrett Browning, 'How Do I Love Thee?'

Emily Dickinson, 'Like Rain It Sounded Till It Curved'

Eugene Field, 'Wynken, Blynken, and Nod'

Felicia Hemans, 'Casabianca'

Francis Ledwidge, 'Thomas McDonagh'

F. W. Harvey, 'Ducks'

Gerard Manley Hopkins, 'Spring'

Gillian Clarke, 'Blue Hydrangeas, September'

Grace Nichols, 'Praise Song for My Mother'

Harold Monro, 'Overheard on a Saltmarsh'

Henry Charles Beeching, 'Going Down Hill on a Bicycle'

Henry Reed, 'Naming of Parts'

Henry Wadsworth Longfellow, 'Psalm of Life'

Hilaire Belloc, 'Tarantella'

Hilaire Belloc, 'The South Country'

Jeane Willie, 'Tea with Aunty Mabel'

Jessie Pope, 'Noise'

John Clare, 'I Love to See the Summer Beaming Forth'

John Clare, 'Little Trotty Wagtail'

John Gillespie Magee, 'High Flight'

John Keats, 'Meg Merrilies'

John Keats, 'To Autumn'

John Masefield, 'Cargoes'

John Masefield, 'Sea Fever'

Joyce Kilmer, 'The House with Nobody in It'

Kenneth H. Ashley, 'Goods Train at Night'

Kenneth Grahame, 'Duck's Ditty'

Langston Hughes, 'Dreams'

Langston Hughes, 'Walkers with the Dawn'

Lemn Sissay, 'Anthem of the North'

Lewis Carroll, 'Jabberwocky'

Marriot Edgar, 'Albert and the Lion'

Maya Angelou, 'Still I Rise'

Ogden Nash, 'Adventures of Isabel'

Percy Bysshe Shelley, 'Ozymandias'

Robert Browning, 'Home Thoughts from Abroad'

Robert Browning, 'How they Brought the Good News from Ghent to Aix'

Robert Burns, 'A Red, Red Rose'

Robert Frost, 'Stopping by Woods on a Snowy Evening'

Robert Frost, 'The Road Not Taken'

Robert Graves, 'Flying Crooked'

Robert Hayden, 'Those Winter Sundays'

Robert Louis Stevenson, 'Windy Nights'

Rudyard Kipling, 'A Smuggler's Song'

Rudyard Kipling, 'If –'

Rudyard Kipling, 'The Way through the Woods'

Rupert Brooke, 'The Old Vicarage, Grantchester'

Rupert Brooke, 'The Soldier'

Samuel Taylor Coleridge, 'Kubla Khan'

Simon Armitage, 'Poundland'

Stevie Smith, 'Not Waving but Drowning'

Stevie Smith, 'The Singing Cat'

Thomas Hardy, 'Weathers'

Walt Whitman, 'O Captain! My Captain!'

Walter de la Mare, 'Some One Came knocking'

Walter de la Mare, 'Silver'

Walter de la Mare, 'The Listeners'

W. B. Yeats, 'The Lake Isle of Innisfree'

W. H. Auden, 'Night Mail'

W. H. Davies, 'Leisure'

Wilfred Owen, 'Dulce et Decorum est'

William Blake, 'The Tyger'

William Ernest Henley, 'Invictus'

William Shakespeare, 'Tell Me Where Is Fancy Bred'

William Shakespeare, 'When Icicles Hang by the Wall'

William Wordsworth, 'I Wandered Lonely as a Cloud'

NOTES AND REFERENCES

Following the example of Francis O'Gorman in his scholarly yet highly readable *Forgetfulness* (Bloomsbury, 2017), I have avoided using superscript numbers in order not to interfere with the reading experience. References for direct and indirect quotations, along with a series of endnotes, appear below. Readers are free to ignore these endnotes: I have used them, to paraphrase Don Paterson, to smuggle in certain technical details and statistics, further examples, and peripheral, but not wholly irrelevant, aperçus and anecdotes. Though it would be a shame to skip these notes entirely, readers can be assured that the main arguments and insights presented in this book make no less sense without them (Paterson, *The Poem: Lyric, Sign Metre*, 2018, p. xvi).

Preface

p. xi   other books published on the same topic: See, for example, the excellent *Reading for Life* and *Is Literature Healthy?* (Philip Davis and Joise Billington respectively) and Kelda Green's equally insightful *Rethinking Therapeutic Reading*.

p. xi   'don't hang grandly together', 'connect in potential meaningful ways': Galen Strawson, *Things That Bother Me* (New York: New York Review of Books, 2018), p. 9.

p. xii   'reading revolution': Jane Davis, 'The Reading Revolution', *Stop What You're Doing and Read This* (London: Vintage, 2011), p. 136.

p. xii   'bringing great writing to life …': Andrea Macmillan, *A Little, Aloud* (London: Chatto & Windus, 2010), p. 12.

p. xii   'one of the most heartening phenomena of our time': Blake Morrison, 'The Reading Cure' *The Guardian* (8 January 2008).

p. xii   to help people with chronic pain: Christopher Dowrick, Josie Billington, Jude Robinson, Andrew Hamer and Clare Williams, 'Get into Reading as an Intervention for Common Mental Health Problems', *Medical Humanities*, vol. 38 (2012), pp. 15–20.

p. xii   to help people with depression: Josie Billington, Anne Louise Humphreys, Andrew Jones and Kate McDonnell, 'A Literature-Based Intervention for People with Chronic Pain', *Arts & Health*, vol. 8, no. 1 (2016), pp. 13–31.

p. xii   'trigger', 'rocket boost', 'reaching levels of emotion …': Philip Davis, *Reading for Life* (Oxford: Oxford University Press, 2020), p. 9.

p. xiii   'extinction rather than evolution': John Sutherland, 'Literature and the Library in the Nineteenth Century', in *The Meaning of the Library: A Cultural History*, edited by Alice Crawford (Princeton, NJ: Princeton University Press, 2015), p. 125.

p. xiv   'my full, true story': Alberto Manguel, *Packing My Library* (New Haven, CT: Yale University Press, 2018), p. 6.

p. xv   'the continuity of self-consciousness …': Eric Matthews, 'Dementia and the Identity of the Person', in *Dementia: Mind, Meaning, and the Person*, edited by Julian Hughes, Stephen Louw and Steven Sabat (Oxford: Oxford University Press, 2005), p. 163.

p. xvi   stringing together the dual narratives: Andrew Solomon, 'Literature about Medicine May Be All That Can Save Us', *The Guardian* (22 April 2016).

p. xvi   'You learn how much grief is about language': Chimamanda Ngozi Adichie, 'Notes on Grief', *The New Yorker* (10 September 2020).

p. xvii   how grief has 'to be done', 'to be expressed': Richard Holloway, *Waiting for the Last Bus* (Edinburgh: Canongate, 2018), p. 138.

p. xvii   'cannot disappear as if it had never been': John Berger, *And Our Faces, My Heart, Brief as Photos* (London: Bloomsbury, 2005), p. 21.

The reading revolution: Shared reading and reading for well-being

p. 2   'doesn't move toward any horizon …': Claude Lucas, *Suerte: L'exclusion Volontaire*, reproduced in Fabrice Guilbaud, 'Working in Prison: Time as Experienced by Inmate-Workers', *Revue Française de Sociologie*, vol. 51, no. 5 (2010), pp. 41–68.

p. 2   Unlike the countless hours spent alone in their cells … According to a recent HM Inspectorate of Prisons report, many prisoners are confined to their cells for long periods of time. For instance, only 14 per cent of prisoners reported spending more than ten hours out of their cell, while 31 per cent reported being locked up for at least twenty-two hours a day, with little to stimulate them. The report concludes, 'When prisoners spend long periods locked in their cells they become frustrated with staff and each other, they are bored and have more time to use illicit substances, and many suffer deteriorating physical and mental health, which can aggravate depression and suicidal feelings' (HM Inspectorate of Prisons, *Life in Prisons: Living Conditions*, 2017, p. 11).

p. 2   a far from passive interpretation of the words on the page: Anne Fadiman, *Ex Libris: Confessions of a Common Reader* (London: Penguin, 2000), p. 107. Fadiman has a wonderful chapter on reading aloud ('Sharing the Mayhem'), and I am indebted to her for introducing me to the writings of Holbrook Jackson, along with Charles Kent's book on Dickens's public readings, *Charles Dickens as a Reader* (Gregg International Publishers, 1971).

p. 3   premised on what it calls 'great' and 'serious' literature: Josie Billington, '"Reading for Life": Prison Reading Groups in Practice and Theory', *Critical Survey*, vol. 23, no. 3 (2011), p. 70.

p. 4   'I read literature as myself, through my own eyes …': Jane Davis, 'Something Real to Carry Home When the Day Is Done', in *English: Shared Futures Essays and Studies*, edited by Robert Eaglestone and Gail Marshall (Cambridge: D. S. Brewer, 2018), p. 212.

p. 6   'creative, social, life-enhancing activity': Billington, 'Reading for Life', p. 70.

p. 6   'Doctors … can't fix a lot of human stuck-ness …' In his fascinating book *Beyond Depression* (Oxford: OUP, 2009), Christopher Dowrick describes situations where hard-pressed GPs, confronted by patients with symptoms not adequately 'explained by physical pathology', sometimes use a diagnosis of depression to impose 'order and understanding in the midst of confusion and chaos'. On such occasions, doctors translate, he suggests, 'raw human suffering' into an illness – something 'therefore treatable' and 'therefore bearable by the doctor' (pp. 113–14). A diagnosis might be convenient for the practitioner, he argues, but it does little to address the needs of patients for whom conventional medicine has little to offer. Dowrick doesn't suggest that standard therapies such as antidepressants are inappropriate responses to emotional turmoil. But he does suggest that we should more readily consider alternatives, responses which help provide patients with a sense of coherence and meaning, responses which, as Josie Billington puts it, recognize that 'the typical causes of depression – loss, trauma, lack – are aspects of experience not susceptible to straightforward correction or cure' (*Is Literature Healthy?*, pp. 2–3).

p. 7   'the mingling of emotions as the work unfolds': Oliver Edwards, *Talking of Books* (London: Heinemann, 1957), p. 20.

p. 8   'has put his ears away in the drawer', and 'all the crescendos, variations of tone …': Friedrich Nietzsche, *Beyond Good and Evil* (Harmondsworth: Penguin, 2003), p. 133.

p. 9   During a reading aloud from *Oliver Twist*: Philip Collins, *Dickens and Crime* (London: Macmillan, 1994), p. 270.

p. 9   'I shall tear myself to pieces': Collins, p. 270.

p. 10   I'm less anxious about getting it wrong … Slips and pratfalls are part of the communal experience of live performance. And happen to the best of us. I think of W. H. Auden reading his poetry aloud to a television studio audience in the 1960s – his stumbling here, his halting there – all the false starts and 'beg your pardons'. And yet, in Auden's case, such a faltering delivery only seems to add to the charm of his recital, endearingly exposing the poet's performative fragility.

p. 10   'to the level of the book': Daniel Pennac, *The Rights of the Reader* (London: Walker Books, 2006), p. 95.

p. 10   'In reading aloud, you are greatly privileged': Holbrook Jackson, *The Anatomy of Bibliomania* (Illinois: University of Illinois Press, 2001), p. 80.

p. 10   'only the writer performs': Fadiman, *Ex Libris*, p. 107.

p. 10   reading aloud is always a collaborative, interpretive process: Fadiman, *Ex Libris*, p. 107.

p. 10   add your voice to their voice: Jackson, *The Anatomy of Bibliomania*, p. 80.

p. 11   'Each year I hoped they'd keep …': Seamus Heaney, 'Blackberry Picking', in *New Selected Poems 1966-1987* (London: Faber and Faber, 2002), p. 130.

p. 12   'ready-made lock-up': John Bayley, 'Reading about Things: Hannibal Goes for the Mail', in *Real Voices: On Reading*, edited by Philip Davis (Basingstoke: Macmillan Press, 1997), p. 180.

p. 13   'the right emotional atmosphere ...', and 'to explore their inner life': Josie Billington, *Is Literature Healthy?* (Oxford: Oxford University Press, 2016), p. 92.

p. 13   'thoughts to be thought ...': Philip Davis and Fiona Magee, *Reading (Arts for Health)* (Bingley: Emerald, 2020), p. 20.

p. 13   One of the most illuminating features of a group reading of Robert Frost's American classic 'The Road Not Taken': Billington, *Is Literature Healthy?*, p. 92.

p. 14   'tries not to make too much': Billington, *Is Literature Healthy?*, p. 93.

p. 15   'she is of course unlikely ever to have children ...': Billington, *Is Literature Healthy?* p. 93.

p. 15   'a powerful sentence in a sensitive area': Davis, *Reading for Life*, p. 75.

p. 15   'opening up hidden lives', 'inner echoes, responses triggered ...': Billington, p. 94.

p. 15   In other (more expressly therapeutic) shared reading settings ... See for example, Josie Billington and Mette Steenberg, 'Literary Reading and Mental-Being', in Donald Kuiken and Arthur Jacobs eds. *Handbook of Empirical Literary Studies* (Berlin: De Gruyter, 2021), pp. 393–420. Josie Billington ed., *Reading and Mental Health* (London: Palgrave, 2019). Eleanor Longden, Philip Davis, Josie Billington, Sofia Lampropoulou, Grace Farrington, Fiona Magee, Erin Walsh and Rhiannon Corcoran, 'Shared Reading: Assessing the Intrinsic Value of a Literature-Based Health Intervention', *Medical Humanities*, vol. 41, no. 2 (2015), pp. 113–20.

p. 15   In one comparative study: Josie Billington, Grace Farrington, Sofia Lampropoulou, Jamie Lingwood, Andrew Jones, James Ledson, Kate McDonnell, Nicky Duirs and Anne-Louise Humphreys, 'A Comparative Study of Cognitive Behavioural Therapy and Shared Reading for Chronic Pain', *Medical Humanities*, vol. 43, no. 3 (2017), pp. 155–65.

p. 17   'notably separate from the suffering she recognizes', 'is a "good thought" ...': Billington et al., 'A Comparative Study of Cognitive Behavioural Therapy and Shared Reading for Chronic Pain', p. 161.

p. 17   'more fully themselves – more fulfilled and absorbed': Josie Billington, Anne Louise Humphreys, Andrew Jones and Kate McDonnell, 'A Literature-Based Intervention for People with Chronic Pain', *Arts & Health*, vol. 8, no. 1 (2016), p. 24.

p. 17   'to recover a whole person, not just an ill one': Billington et al., 'A Comparative Study', p. 163.

p. 18   shared reading responds to so much human strife and struggle: Davis, *Reading for Life*, p. 11.

p. 18   'so that everyone can experience ...': The Reader Organisation, 'Project Update and FAQS: June 2019', https://www.thereader.org.uk/project-update-and-faqs-june-2019.

p. 18   'mood-busting books', and 'recommended by other readers to help lift your mood': The Reading Agency, 'Reading Well: Mood-Boosting Books, 2024', https://reading-well.org.uk/books/mood-boosting-books.

p. 19   'towards problem solving...': Sarah Jack and Kevin Ronan, 'Bibliotherapy: Practice
          and Research', *School Psychology International*, vol. 29, no. 2 (2008), p. 164.

p. 19   The term 'bibliotherapy' was coined: Samuel McChord Crothers, 'A Literary
          Clinic', *The Atlantic*, vol. 118, no. 3 (1916), pp. 291–301.

p. 19   'During the last year I have been working up ...', and 'From my point of view, a
          book is a literary prescription ...': McChord Crothers, 'A Literary Clinic', p. 292.

p. 19   'I was sorry because I wished to discuss with him ...': McChord Crothers, 'A
          Literary Clinic', p. 301.

p. 19   The scheme was devised in 2003: Neil Frude, 'Book Prescriptions – A Strategy
          for Delivering Psychological Treatment in the Primary Care Setting', *The Mental
          Health Review*, vol. 10, no. 4 (2005), pp. 30–3.

p. 20   'a growing awareness of the desirability of providing ...': Frude, 'Book
          Prescriptions', p. 30.

p. 20   'over 2.6 million Reading Well books have been borrowed ...': The Reading
          Agency, 'Books That Offer Hope, March 2021' (Reading-Well, 2021).

p. 20   'As an "off-the-peg" treatment ...': Frude, 'Book Prescriptions', p. 32.

p. 21   'Too often the prescribed "literature" in local libraries ...': Blake Morrison, 'The
          Reading Cure', *The Guardian* (8 January 2008).

p. 21   'selected with specific therapeutic outcomes in mind', 'relevance to the human
          condition': Ellie Gray, *Making Sense of Mental Health Difficulties through Live
          Reading: An Interpretative Phenomenological Analysis of the Experience of Being in
          a Reader Group* (Liverpool: University of Liverpool, 2013), p. 3.

p. 21   In their excellent book: Sarah McNichol and Liz Brewster, *Bibliotherapy*
          (London: Routledge, 2018).

p. 22   In one of my favourite studies: Cristina Deberti Martins, 'Bibliotherapy in
          Uruguay: A Case Study of the Mario Benedetti Library for Patients Dealing with
          Substance Abuse', in *Bibliotherapy*, edited by Sarah McNichol and Liz Brewster
          (London: Facet, 2018), pp. 129–40.

p. 22   'left them with feelings of frustration ...': Martins, 'Bibliotherapy in Uruguay',
          p. 135.

p. 22   'they feel disconnected from their past ...', 'everyday life revolves around getting
          the substance ...': Martins, 'Bibliotherapy in Uruguay', p. 138.

p. 23   Reading and discussing poetry with others provided them with a private
          sanctuary: Martins, 'Bibliotherapy in Uruguay', p. 138.

p. 24   'seemed to have nothing left to live for': John Stuart Mill, *Autobiography*
          (London: Oxford University Press, 1958), p. 113.

p. 24   'he was not the physician who could heal it': Mill, *Autobiography*, p. 115.

p. 24   'What made Wordsworth's poems a medicine ...': Mill, *Autobiography*, p. 125.

p. 25   'had felt that the first freshness ...': Mill, *Autobiography*, p. 126.

p. 25   'but poetry of deeper and loftier feeling ...': Mill, *Autobiography*, p. 126.

p. 25   'the purest and best form of bibliotherapy': Ella Berthoud and Susan Elderkin,
          The Novel Cure (Edinburgh: Canongate, 2015), p. 1.

p. 26   'Sometimes it's the story that charms ...': Berthoud and Elderkin, *The Novel
          Cure*, p. 1.

p. 26   'Read it for the ease with which the words will tumble out': Berthoud and
           Elderkin, *The Novel Cure*, p. 96.

p. 26   'the way it drives you to agree or disagree with the authors' choices': Gavin
           Francis, 'The Novel Cure by Susan Elderkin and Ella Berthoud – Review', *The
           Guardian* (18 September 2013).

p. 26   'real healing power for readers': Serena Cacchioli, 'The Healing Power of
           Books: The Novel Cure as a Culturally Tailored Literary Experiment', *Reading
           Today* (2018), p. 147.

p. 26   'does not distinguish between emotional and physical pain': Francis, 'The Novel
           Cure by Susan Elderkin and Ella Berthoud – Review'.

p. 27   an experience she elegantly describes in the New Yorker: Ceridwen Dovey, 'Can
           Reading Make You Happier?' *The New Yorker* (9 June 2015).

p. 27   'I am worried about having no spiritual resources …': Dovey, 'Can Reading Make
           You Happier?'.

p. 29   'ability to withstand terrible grief untested', 'are still nebulous …', and 'In a secular
           age …': Dovey, 'Can Reading Make You Happier?'.

p. 30   'troubling questions', 'what's lost when a bookshelf is repurposed …', 'to find out
           what happens next …': Leah Price, 'When Doctors Prescribe Books to Heal the
           Mind', *The Boston Globe* (22 December 2013).

p. 30   'project of making literature more usable to lay readers …': Leah Price,
           'Bibliotherapy and Human Flourishing', in *Literary Studies and Human
           Flourishing*, edited by James English and Heather Love (Oxford: Oxford
           University Press, 2023), p. 32.

p. 30   'instead of inciting readers to rage …': Price, 'Bibliotherapy and Human
           Flourishing', p. 30.

p. 31   'turns and nuances and telling details': Philip Davis, *Reading for Life*, p. 8.

p. 31   'A public library system suffering even more drastic budget cuts …': Leah Price,
           *What We Talk about When We Talk about Books: The History and Future of
           Reading* (New York: Basic Books, 2019), p. 120.

p. 31   'solves no problems and saves no souls': Derek Attridge, *The Singularity of
           Literature* (London: Routledge, 2004), p. 5.

p. 31   'fourth-rate journals': Raymond Tallis cited in Blake Morrison, 'The Reading
           Cure', *The Guardian* (8 January 2008).

p. 31   Such meta-analysis studies have shown … See, for example, Paul Montgomery
           and Kathryn Maunders, 'The Effectiveness of Creative Bibliotherapy for
           Internalizing, Externalizing, and Prosocial Behaviors in Children: A Systematic
           Review', *Children and Youth Services Review*, vol. 55 (2015), pp. 37–47; Calla
           Glavin and Paul Montgomery, 'Creative Bibliotherapy for Post-Traumatic Stress
           Disorder (PTSD): A Systematic Review', *Journal of Poetry Therapy*, vol. 30, no. 2
           (2017), pp. 95–107.

p. 32   creative bibliotherapy and shared reading can help reduce the symptoms: Sara
           James and Juliane Römhild, 'Practising Creative Bibliotherapy Down
           Under: Understanding Diverse Approaches to Literature as Therapy', *Journal of
           Poetry Therapy*, vol. 37, no. 3 (2023), pp. 173–84.

p. 32   The kinds of emotive, aesthetic texts: Deborah Dysart-Gale, 'Lost in Translation: Bibliotherapy and Evidence-Based Medicine', *Journal of Medical Humanities* vol. 28, no. 1 (2008), p. 35.

p. 32   'may never be able to capture' the kind and quantity of data that 'scientists hunger for': Jonathan Bate and Andrew Schuman, 'Books do Furnish a Mind: The Art and Science of Bibliotherapy', *The Lancet*, vol. 387, no. 10020 (2016), p. 743.

p. 32   'speaks volumes for those who care to listen': Bate and Schuman, 'Books do Furnish a Mind', p. 743.

What have libraries ever done for us?
In defence of the public library system

p. 33   the Sieghart report, an independent review on the future of public libraries: William Sieghart, *Independent Library Report for England* (London: Department for Culture, Media and Sport, 2014).

p. 34   promising to implement its key recommendations ... The Sieghart Review's key recommendations for central government were: to provide funding to increase Wi-Fi access in public libraries, to establish a council-led library task force charged with creating a national digital library network and (more nebulously) to have greater cross-government support for libraries. Although well-meaning and generally well-received, the Sieghart Review was criticized by some library commentators and sections of the media who described it as a fudge, a report which failed to take into account the immediately pressing context of library cuts and closures.

p. 34   'a cherished part of our cultural heritage ...': Edward Vaizey, 'Written Statement made by: The Minister of State for Culture and the Digital Economy on 18 Dec 2014' (London, Department for Culture Media and Sport, 2014).

p. 35   'to follow the stranger whithersoever he would go': Edgar Allan Poe, *Tales of Mystery and Imagination* (London: Everyman, 1993), p. 112.

p. 35   'the love of libraries, like other loves, must be learnt': Alberto Manguel, *The Library at Night* (New Haven, CT: Yale University Press, 2006), p. 4.

p. 36   'a great library': William Gass, *Life Sentences: Literary Judgments and Accounts* (New York: Knopf, 2012), p. 15.

p. 37   'During the half hour I was in or near it ...': John Redwood, 'A Visit to a Library', *John Redwood's Diary* (5 April 2011).

p. 39   'totally unacceptable': BBC, 'Protesters stage overnight sit-in at New Cross library', *BBC News* (6 February 2011).

p. 39   'to exempt libraries from cuts ...': Keith Mitchell, Letter to the *Guardian* (31 January 2011). In his letter, Mitchell was responding to a speech given by Philip Pullman to an Oxfordshire library campaigners' meeting, in which the celebrated author criticized Oxfordshire County Council's decision to close a number of its libraries.

p. 40   'structural reminder of civic values': Anne Goulding, *Public Libraries in the 21st Century: Defining Services and Debating the Future* (London: Routledge, 2016), p. 11.

p. 43   heightens children's sensitivity to language … Numerous studies have demonstrated how reading aloud to children fosters early literacy (for just a few examples, see Dolores Durkin, *Teaching Young Children to Read* (Boston, MA: Allyn and Bacon, 1980); Hollis Scarborough and Wanda Dobrich, 'On the Efficacy of Reading to Pre-Schoolers', *Developmental Review*, vol. 14, no. 3 (1994), pp. 245–302; Monique Sénéchal and Jo-Anne LeFevre, 'Parental Involvement in the Development of Children's Reading Skill: A Five-Year Longitudinal study', *Child Development*, vol. 73, no. 2 (2002), pp. 445–60). In her classic treatise on early reading, *Beginning to Read* (Cambridge, MA: MIT Press, 1990), Marilyn Adams describes reading aloud to children as 'the most important activity for building the knowledge and skills eventually required for reading' (p. 86). Reading accounts for approximately a third of a child's vocabulary acquisition and hence leads to 'substantial and permanent learning and greater school achievement' (Donna Celano and Susan Neuman, *The Role of Public Libraries in Children's Literacy Development* (Pennsylvania, PA: Pennsylvania Library Association, 2001), p. 9). Equally important, though I think its significance is sometimes overlooked in the research literature, is the enjoyment to be had in reading aloud, which helps engender positive feelings towards books and the learning environment.

p. 43   providing parents who might struggle with reading: Elisabeth Duursma, Marilyn Augustyn and Barry Zuckerman, 'Reading Aloud to Children: The Evidence', *Archives of Disease in Childhood*, vol. 93, no. 7 (2008), pp. 554–7.

p. 43   'can sometimes have a whiff of do-goodery about them': Terence Blacker, 'Why Books Are a Lifeline for Prisoners', *Independent* (2 April 2014).

p. 44   Right from the beginning, prior to the Public Libraries Act of 1850 … The potted history of the British public library that follows here is based on two excellent sources: Thomas Kelly, *Books for the People: An Illustrated History of the British Public Library* (London: André Deutsch, 1977), and Nick Moore, 'Public Library Trends', *Cultural Trends*, vol. 13, no. 1 (2004), pp. 27–57.

p. 45   'Free libraries are "god-sends" to the town loafer …': M. D. O'Brien, 'Free Libraries', in *A Plea for Liberty*, edited by Thomas Mackay (New York: Murray, 1891), p. 829.

p. 45   'There a few doors which a golden key will not unlock': Kelly, *An Illustrated History of the British Public Library*, 92.

p. 46   with the decade between 1965 and 1975 being described as its 'golden age': Moore, 'Public Library Trends', p. 41.

p. 46   which sought to introduce market mechanisms to the running of the library: Frank Webster, *Theories of the Information Society* (London: Routledge, 1995), p. 222.

p. 46   All of which calls to mind that ardent champion of the public library, Alan
         Bennett: Alan Bennett, 'What I Did in 2015', *London Review of Books* (7 January 2016).

p. 47   many libraries had been shut down and were continuing to close: Chartered
         Institute of Public Finance and Accountancy (CIPFA), *Public Library Statistics
         2015/16.*

p. 47   'Books are available for free …': John McTernan, 'Don't Mourn the Loss of
         Libraries – The Internet Has Made Them Obsolete', *The Telegraph* (29 March
         2016). Reading McTernan's article online, I was gratified to note that, for all the
         loyalty of his fan base, his argument appeared to cut little ice with his *Telegraph*
         audience: when asked in an interactive online survey whether they lamented the
         decline of libraries ('Yes – we're losing our cultural foundations / No – technology
         is making them less useful'), 75 per cent of readers answered in the affirmative.

p. 48   Public libraries – and I suspect this is something librarians have known
         all along – are 'therapeutic landscapes': Wilbert Gesler, 'Therapeutic
         Landscapes: Medical Issues in Light of the New Cultural Geography', *Social
         Science & Medicine*, vol. 34, no. 7 (1992), pp. 735–46.

p. 48   a growing body of research has demonstrated the positive impact that library
         environments have on people's health … Most of the research evaluating the
         public library system tends to be qualitative in nature. But for all the challenges
         of evaluating public libraries in quantitative monetary terms, there have been
         a number of determined attempts to do so. One noteworthy example – a study
         commissioned by Arts Council England (Simetrica, *The Health and Wellbeing
         Benefits of Public Libraries* (2015)) – aimed to quantify the contribution that
         public libraries make to public health in terms of financial savings. Using a
         contingent valuation approach, a method of analysis that assesses people's
         willingness to pay for non-market services, the research examined the responses
         of 2,000 participants who were surveyed about their library (and non-library)
         use. The research also combed through pre-existing datasets, including national
         survey data that detailed people's general health, lifestyle choices and other
         demographic determinants of well-being. The aggregate data revealed that health
         and subjective well-being, as well as higher life satisfaction, were associated with
         regular library use. Based on such a positive correlation, the authors of the study
         extrapolated that the impact of library services on general health would save the
         exchequer £748.1 million per year.

p. 48   Brewster has shown how the library space was often a lifeline for people recovering
         from mental health problems: Liz Brewster, 'The Public Library as Therapeutic
         Landscape: A Qualitative Case Study', *Health & Place*, vol. 26 (2014), pp. 94–9.

p. 49   libraries are not seen as controlling, regulating spaces: Sarah Johnsen, Paul Cloke
         and Jon May, 'Day Centres for Homeless People: Spaces of Care or Fear?', *Social
         & Cultural Geography* vol. 6, no. 6 (2005), pp. 787–811.

p. 49   In a study that examined homeless men's use of the public library: Darrin
         Hodgetts, Ottilie Stolte, Kerry Chamberlain, Alan Radley, Linda Nikora, Eci
         Nabalarua and Shiloh Groot, 'A Trip to the Library: Homelessness and Social
         Inclusion', *Social & Cultural Geography*, vol. 9, no. 8 (2008), pp. 933–53.

p. 49   'to read books and do what everyone else uses the library for …': Hodgetts et al.,
         'A Trip to the Library', p. 941.

p. 49   the 'last thing on earth' they wanted to do was to 'have a chat with
         somebody': Brewster, 'The Public Library as Therapeutic Landscape', p. 97.

p. 50   a kind of secular cathedral inhabited by the lone scholar: Anne Goulding, 'The
         Rise, Fall and Rise of the British Public Library Building', in *17th BOBCATSSS
         Symposium* (January 2009), pp. 28–39.

p. 50   the 'great unsold truth' of modern public libraries: Bella Bathurst, 'The Secret Lives
         of Libraries', in *The Library Book*, edited by Rebecca Gray (London: Profile Books,
         2012), p. 76.

p. 50   Writing about the experience of writing his first book: Alfred Kazin, *New York
         Jew* (Syracuse: Syracuse University Press, 1996), p. 7.

p. 51   For when a library closes, what users report missing most of all: Richard
         Usherwood, Bob Proctor and Gill Sobczyk, 'What Happens When a Public Library
         Service Closes Down?' *Library Management*, vol. 18, no. 1 (1997), pp. 59–64.

p. 51   To close any library is to create both 'a physical and social gap in the
         community': Anne Goulding, 'The Public Library: A Successful Public Space?', in
         Spaces, Speciality and Technology, edited by Phil Turner and Elisabeth Davenport
         (AA Dordrecht, the Netherlands: Springer, 2005), p. 63.

p. 51   'I don't know of anything more disheartening than the sight of a shut down
         library': Charles Simic, 'A Country without Libraries', *New York Review of Books* (18
         May 2011).

p. 52   'What can be found there has undone dictators and tyrants': Doris Lessing,
         'Doris Lessing', in *The Pleasure of Reading*, edited by Antonia Fraser
         (London: Bloomsbury, 1992), p. 47.

p. 52   'people who have access to good libraries …': Lessing, 'Doris Lessing', p. 47.

p. 52   'an alternative world, a way of living apart': Jon Cook, 'Lorna Sage', *The Guardian*
         (13 January, 2001).

Reawakening the mind: Poetry and the new culture of dementia care

p. 55   rebelling, as he puts it: Alberto Manguel, 'Some Thoughts About Thinking',
         Cognitive and Behavorial Neurology, vol. 28, no. 2 (2015), p. 43.

P. 55   'I was unable to mouth the words …': Manguel, 'Some Thoughts', p. 43.

p. 56   'there is something undeniably important …': Rafael Campo, *The Healing Art: A
         Doctor's Black Bag of Poetry* (New York: WW Norton, 2003), p. 2.

p. 57   'surviving "self" to the fore': Oliver Sacks, *Musicophilia* (London: Picador, 2011),
         p. 382.

p. 57   dementia is defined as a chronic: Tom Dening and Malarvizhi Babu Sandilyan,
         'Dementia: Definitions and Types', *Nursing Standard*, vol. 29, no. 37 (2015), p. 38.

p. 57   Although the cause of dementia is not fully known: Tom Dening and Malarvizhi Babu Sandilyan, 'Dementia', p. 38.

p. 58   which accounts for approximately 75 per cent of all cases: Dening and Sandilyan, 'Dementia', p. 39.

p. 58   pharmaceutical remedies have had little impact: Tom Dening and Malarvizhi Babu Sandilyan, 'Medical Treatment and Management of Patients with Dementia', *Nursing Standard*, vol. 29, no. 45 (2015), p. 44.

p. 58   'Prescribed disengagement®': Kate Swaffer, *What the Hell Happened to My Brain? Living Beyond Dementia* (London: Jessica Kingsley, 2016), p. 157.

p. 58   'Dementia is the only disease or condition I know of…', 'Having dementia does not mean you have to give up …', and 'Dementia may well be a terminal illness …': Kate Swaffer, 'Dementia and Prescribed Disengagement', *Dementia*, vol. 14, no. 1 (2015), p. 4.

p. 59   Yet, as the late, great Tom Kitwood argued: Tom Kitwood, *Dementia Reconsidered: The Person Comes First* (Berkshire: Open University Press, 1997).

p. 59   are due to pathological changes in the brain: Tom Kitwood, 'Brain, Mind and Dementia: With Particular Reference to Alzheimer's Disease', *Ageing and Society*, vol. 9, no. 1 (1989), p. 13.

p. 59   Some are due to what he called 'malignant social psychology': Tom Kitwood and Kathleen Bredin, 'Towards a Theory of Dementia Care', *Ageing and Society*, vol. 12, no. 3 (1992), p. 271. For a complete account of the ways in which the social environment both positively and negatively affects the person with dementia, as well as an introduction to Kitwood's theories more generally, see his seminal and highly readable *Dementia Reconsidered: The Person Comes First*.

p. 59   'Tom always had to battle with the establishment …': Bob Woods, 'Editorial. The Legacy of Kitwood. Professor Tom Kitwood 1937–1998', *Aging & Mental Health*, vol. 3, no. 1 (1999), p. 6.

p. 60   given rise to a flourishing of activities: Hannah Zeilig, John Killick and Chris Fox, 'The Participative Arts for People Living with a Dementia: A Critical Review', *International Journal of Ageing and Later Life*, vol. 9, no. 1 (2014), pp. 7–34. Besides helping to maintain personhood and personal identity, psychosocial approaches to dementia care have also been shown to reduce dependency on antipsychotic medication prescribed to manage so-called 'challenging behaviours' (aggression, agitation, hallucinations, etc.) in people with dementia.

p. 60   as Oliver Sacks has shown: Oliver Sacks, *Musicophilia* (London: Picador, 2011).

p. 60   it's not unreasonable to suggest we also possess a poetic memory … Discussing the mnemonic power of poetry in his compendious *The Poem: Lyric, Sign, Metre* (London: Faber, 2018), the poet Don Paterson describes the poem as 'a little machine for remembering itself' (itself a memorable description). The memory and the acquisition of a poem, Paterson argues, are 'one of the same thing':

> The memory of a symphony, painting, film or novel, however vivid, is no more than that: just a memory, or at best a very partial recovery … A remembered story perhaps remains more closely the story - but only its structure remains intact, not its form of words. But if you remember a poem, you possess it

wholly. To recall a poem is the poem; the poem has become, quite literally, part of your being. (p. 10)

Paterson doesn't specifically address the issue of the persistence of poetic memory in the context of cognitive decline, locating poetry's general ability to transcend the constraints of human memory in three formal characteristics: poetry as brief speech, patterned speech and original speech. One reason why the ability to respond to poetry remains preserved in people with dementia is that poetic memory might be partially coextensive with musical memory. Several experimental studies have shown how parts of the brain associated with musical memory are preserved in individuals with dementia – even in very late stages of the syndrome. The precise mechanisms by which it is spared in people with dementia, however, are not fully understood and remain somewhat speculative. For an in-depth discussion of musical and poetic memories respectively, see Matthew Schulkind, 'Is Memory for Music Special?' (*Annals of the New York Academy of Sciences*, vol. 1169, no. 1 (2009), pp. 216–24), and Nigel Fabb, *What Is Poetry? Language and Memory in the Poems of the World* (Cambridge: Cambridge University Press, 2015), pp. 171–91.

p. 62   conditions there … were more like those witheringly described in the classic sociological critiques of residential care in the 1950s and 1960s … I am thinking here of Peter Townsend's and Michael Meacher's famous studies, *The Last Refuge* and *Taken for a Ride*. These two seminal critiques were the first of their kind to provide extensive ethnographic accounts of the experiences of older people living in institutional care following the UK's 1948 National Assistance Act, which compelled local authorities to provide care and accommodation for anyone 'substantially handicapped by illness, injury or cognitive deformity'. Although focusing on different contexts (Townsend's study reported on care homes in the 1950s, while Meacher's examined homes in the 1960s), both studies exposed, often in unforgettable detail, the indignities, enduring tribulations and crippling lack of self-determination experienced by people living in residential care. What also comes through in these accounts is the utter meaninglessness of the lives of residents subject to stultifying routines run principally for the benefit of the institution. As Meacher memorably put it: 'above everything else lies the pall of hours to be lived through with no obvious satisfactory purpose left'.

p. 63   'Miracle on St David's Day': Gillian Clarke, 'Miracle on St David's Day', in *Collected Poems* (Manchester: Carcanet, 1997), p. 36.

p. 65   the lines acting, in Oliver Sacks' phrase, as a kind of 'Proustian mnemonic': Sacks, *Musicophilia*, p. 380.

p. 65   I recalled comments made by the gerontologist Henk Loning: Douwe Draaisma, *The Nostalgia Factory: Memory, Time and Ageing* (New Haven: Yale University Press, 2013), pp. 97–8.

p. 68   I wondered whether, somewhat fancifully … In his various encounters with neurologically impaired patients, Oliver Sacks and his colleagues often attempted to devise ways of maintaining the curative effects brought about by the use of more unorthodox (i.e. non-medical) interventions, music therapy especially. In his book of case studies, *An Anthropologist on Mars* (London: Picador, 2012), for example, Sacks recounts the case of Greg, a highly musical and amnesiac patient who, reduced to a near-permanent state of vacancy and disorientation by a brain tumour, would come to himself whenever he listened to or played music, shedding in the process his lethargy and indifference and evincing great feeling and connectedness. This being so, would it not be possible, Sacks speculated, to embed certain specific pieces of information in songs (to which Greg was receptive) – or even compose songs with specially penned lyrics – as a means of helping him remember important details and achieve a more enduring therapeutic response?

Ingenious as it was, the proposed scheme was unsuccessful: Greg would relapse into his original, impaired state. As Sacks later records in *Musicophilia*, there was no possibility of any carry-over from implicit memory (which permits the unconscious performance of procedural actions) to explicit memory, and consequently no possibility of practically implementing a musical-mnemonic framework that would have assisted Greg with routine thinking and living.

p. 69 harnesses the 'very foundational, subcortical levels of the brain': Sacks, *Musicophilia*, p. 382.

p. 69 'intoxicating' influence of metre: Samuel Taylor Coleridge, *Biographia Literaria: Biographical Sketches of My Literary Life and Opinions* (London: Everyman, 1997), p. 220. In her intriguing article 'Coleridge and the Pleasures of Verse', (*Studies in Romanticism*, vol. 40, no. 4 (2001), pp. 547–69), Anya Taylor makes the claim that whereas metre for Coleridge was an 'upper', a stimulant to excitement, for Wordsworth, his close friend and collaborator, metre was a 'downer', a means of managing and controlling emotions. This is not to suggest that the metrical design of Wordsworth's poetry isn't in any way conducive to arousal and agitation, but that, for Wordsworth, the essential purpose of metre was 'to soothe rather than to exhilarate'.

There's something in this. I have often noticed the calming, steadying influence that many of Wordsworth's poems – 'The Solitary Reaper', 'I Wandered Lonely as a Cloud' and 'A Slumber did my Spirit Seal' – have had on listeners, inducing in them a sleepy torpor ... It used to irritate me if anyone nodded off during my recitals – I wanted my reading to function as a spur, not as a sedative – until one care worker pointed out that, with respect to settling anxious residents, poetry-induced slumber was far more preferable to sedation by antipsychotic medication.

p. 69 'the vivacity and susceptibility of the general feelings ...': Coleridge, *Biographia Literaria*, p. 220.

p. 70 'are charged with precise lexical sense ...': David Constantine, *Poetry: The Literary Agenda* (Oxford: Oxford University Press, 2013), p. 58.

p. 70 'The musical and pictorial powers of the right brain ...': Frederick Turner and Ernst Pöppel, 'The Neural Lyre: Poetic Metre, the Brain and Time', *Poetry*, vol. 142, no. 5 (1983), p. 306.

p. 70   'poetry gives both sides of our brain …': Salman Akhtar, 'A Bit of Prose about
         Poetry', *International Journal of Applied Psychoanalytic Studies*, vol. 5, no. 2
         (2008), p. 92.

p. 71   'the brain's capacities for self-reward' and 'nicely fulfills …': Turner and Pöppel,
         'The Neural Lyre', p. 306.

p. 71   quite another to claim that our neural system is in perfect accord: Alan Holder,
         Rethinking Meter: A New Approach to the Verse Line (Lewisburg, PA: Bucknell
         University Press, 1995), p. 69.

p. 71   An illustrative example is Noreen O'Sullivan and colleagues' (2015) study: Noreen
         O'Sullivan, Philip Davis, Josie Billington, Victorina Gonzalez-Diaz and Rhiannon
         Corcoran, '"Shall I Compare Thee": The Neural Basis of Literary Awareness, and
         Its Benefits to Cognition', *Cortex*, vol. 73 (2015), pp. 144–57.

p. 73   scourge of what he calls 'neuromania': Raymond Tallis, *Aping Mankind*
         (London: Routledge, 2016).

p. 74   functional neuroimaging research contributes relatively little to our
         understanding and experience of poetry … The poet Dan Paterson argues that,
         though his colleagues refer to brain imaging approaches as 'neurobollocks',
         his preference is for any material explanation of poetic experience – no matter
         how outlandish or reductive. Despite 'the self-justifying pseudo-science
         of much of its methodology', a neuroscientific approach is, he observes,
         better than one 'predicated on fairies, pixies, God, inscrutable intercessors,
         sympathetic magic, or dark and unseen forces. In its dogged refusal to supply
         adequate descriptions of intermediary mechanism, critical theory can sound
         as much of a mysterian cult as theology' (*The Poem: Lyric, Sign, Metre*, p. 106).

p. 76   Conceived by the Dutch psychologist Bère Miesen: Bère Miesen and Gemma
         Jones, 'The Alzheimer Café Concept: A Response to the Trauma, Drama and
         Tragedy of Dementia', in *Caregiving in Dementia: Research and Applications 3*,
         edited by Gemma Jones and Bère Miesen (Hove: Brunner Routledge, 2004), pp.
         307–34.

p. 76   breaking free from the stigma: Miesen and Jones, 'The Alzheimer Café
         Concept'.

p. 78   to 'bloom' with symbol and allusion: John Killick, *You are Words: Dementia
         Poems* (London: Hawker Publications, 2008), p. 7.

p. 78   'the natural language of those with dementia is poetry': Killick, *You are
         Words*, p. 7.

p. 78   'I make it clear … they can talk about anything …': John Killick, 'Giving
         Voice: Writing Poetry', in *Creativity and Communication in Persons with
         Dementia: A Practical Guide*, edited by Claire Craig and John Killick
         (London: Jessica Kingsley, 2012), p. 45.

p. 79   In a postscript to *You Are Words*: Killick, *You Are Words*, p. 72.

p. 80   'As can be imagined, reactions to the poems …': Killick, 'Giving Voice: Writing
         Poetry', p. 46.

p. 80   'language has acknowledged, has given shelter to …': John Berger, *And Our Faces,
         My Heart, Brief as Photos* (London: Bloomsbury, 2005), p. 21.

p. 80   'that their words are being taken seriously', 'that it is worth communicating with people with dementia': Killick, 'Giving Voice: Writing Poetry', p. 46.

The enduring self: A journal

p. 84   Although dementia has affected his speech: In *Conversations with an Alzheimer's Patient* (Cambridge: Cambridge University Press, 1994), a linguistic study of dementia discourse, Heidi Hamilton refers to three characteristic stages of Alzheimer's disease in terms of communicative decline: early or mild, middle or moderate, and late or severe. The early stage involves difficulties with word-finding and object naming – but is not so marked that problems can't be covered up by certain linguistic strategies. The middle stage is marked by increased naming difficulties, problems maintaining meaningful conversation and reduced interactivity. The late stage is characterized by a 'general lack of communication and possibly even lack of awareness that another person is present' (11).

p. 84   I share 'their associations, their public meanings': Jane Miller, *Crazy Age* (London: Hachette, 2010), p. 47.

p. 86   they are safe, highly managed places: Stephen Fineman, *Organizing Age* (Oxford: Oxford University Press, 2011) p. 127.

p. 87   'Nothing in the world can rob us of the power to say "I"': Simone Weil, *Simone Weil: An Anthology*, edited by Siân Miles (Harmondsworth: Penguin, 2005), p. 99.

p. 87   The last words of the great satirist Jonathan Swift: Irvin Ehrenpreis, *The Personality of Jonathan Swift* (Cambridge, MA: Harvard University Press, 1958), p. 147.

p. 87   they will have 'displayed an intact self': Steven Sabat and Rom Harré, 'The Construction and Deconstruction of Self in Alzheimer's Disease', *Ageing & Society*, vol. 12, no. 4 (1992), p. 447.

p. 88   'a patient [with severe dementia] may have the capacity …': Michael Luntley, 'Keeping Track, Autobiography, and the Conditions for Self-Erosion', in *Dementia: Mind, Meaning, and the Person*, edited by Julian Hughes, Stephen Louw and Steven Sabat (Oxford: Oxford University Press, 2005), p. 106.

p. 89   In his editorial notes on 'If–': Craig Raine, 'Introduction' to *Kipling: Selected Poetry*, edited by Craig Raine (Harmondsworth: Penguin, 2001), p. xxvi.

p. 90   John Bayley's biography of his wife, the novelist and philosopher Iris Murdoch: John Bayley, *Iris* (London: Duckworth Overlook, 2012).

p. 90   'we are still part of each other': Bayley, *Iris*, p. 249.

p. 90   'Iris not only smiled …': Bayley, *Iris*, p. 249.

p. 90   'For someone who had been accustomed not so much to read books …': Bayley, *Iris*, p. 249.

p. 91   'not merely to uncover, to bring out deficits …': Oliver Sacks, *The Man Who Mistook His Wife for a Hat* (London: Picador, 2015), pp. 171–2.

p. 91   Testing, moreover, is often self-fulfilling … The enduring capacities and character
            of the person with dementia elude cognitive assessments. In shining a light on
            what is lost, testing fails to show the things that people can still do. ('You keep
            telling me what's been lost, and I keep telling you something remains', says the
            narrator of Michael Ignatieff's novel, *Scar Tissue*, as he discusses his mother's
            dementia test results with her doctor.) Testing provides little insight into the
            personal reality of living with dementia, the various ways in which individuals,
            with or without support, are able to adapt and help themselves. Surely what
            counts is what the person does in the world?

p. 94   John Bayley likened the talk between himself and Iris to 'underwater
            sonar': Bayley, *Iris*, p. 249.

p. 99   'all the poetic cliches': Al Alvarez, *Pondlife* (London: Bloomsbury, 2013), p. 61.

p. 101   comprised as they are of phonemes that harness the standard sound patterns
            of English: Marnie Parsons, *Touch Monkeys: Nonsense Strategies for Reading
            Twentieth-Century Poetry* (Toronto: University of Toronto Press, 1994), p. 3.

p. 104   'touched by the mild boredom of order': Walter Benjamin, 'Unpacking My
            Library: A Talk about Book Collecting', in *Illuminations*, edited by Hannah
            Arendt (San Diego, CA: Harcourt, Brace & World, 1968), p. 59.

p. 105   Like all intellectuals, he evidently read with a pencil in his hand … I refer here
            to George Steiner's wry definition: 'The intellectual is, quite simply, a human
            being who has a pencil in his or her hand when reading a book' (*No Passion
            Spent: Essays, 1978–1996* (London: Faber, 1996), p. 11).

p. 105   'A life that has been well lived and a shared sense of happiness and
            accomplishment …': Sherwin Nuland, *How We Die: Reflections on Life's Final
            Chapter* (New York: Vintage, 1994), p. 105.

April notebook: A death in the family

p. 123   'to some still undiscovered and undefined "other side"': Edwidge Danticat,
            The Art of Death: Writing the Final Story (Minneapolis, MN: Graywolf Press,
            2020), p. 7.

p. 126   How can I step into May: David Grossman, *Falling Out of Time* (London: Vintage,
            2014), p. 139.

p. 126   'the inverse of life': Grossman, *Falling Out of Time,* p. 14.

p. 126   'It is well known that mourners often get the illness …': Lily Pincus, *Death and the
            Family: The Importance of Mourning* (London: Faber & Faber, 1997), p. 121.

p. 127   'Snow, a real snowstorm over Paris; strange …': Roland Barthes, *Mourning Diary*
            (London: Notting Hill Editions, 2011), p. 93.

p. 129   'stable banality of routine living': Aleksandar Hemon, *The Book of My Lives*
            (London: Macmillan, 2013), p. 202.

p. 129   only that in no way has he ceased to exist: Julian Barnes, *Levels of Life* (London:
            Penguin Random House, 2013), p. 102

p. 130   But as Barthes suggests: Barthes, *Mouring Diary*, p. 68.

p. 132   To which quests were you yoked?: Euripedes (trans. Richard Aldington), *Alcestis* (London: Chatto & Windus, 1930), p. 30.

p. 133   'You don't come out of it like a train …': Julian Barnes, *Levels of Life* (London: Vintage, 2013), p. 114.

p. 133   'comforting messages received from the other realm': Edward Parnell, *Ghostland* (London: William Collins, 2019), pp. 107–8.

p. 133   'Where are the snakes with you?': Parnell, *Ghostland*, p. 108.

p. 134   'as solid evidence of an afterlife …': Parnell, *Ghostland*, p. 109.

p. 134   'Not in the darkened rooms …': Roy Fuller, 'Ghost Voice' in *New and Collected Poems* (London: Secker & Warburg, 1985), p. 438.

p. 136   'A Waiting Room in August': Julia Darling, 'A Waiting Room in August', in Julia Darling, Incredible, Miraculous: *The Collected Poems of Julia Darling*, edited by Bev Robinson (Todmorden: Arc Publications, 2015), p. 24.

p. 136   What's it like to die?: Grossman, *Falling Out of Time*, p. 130.

p. 138   'no sooner has she departed …': Barthes, *Mouring Diary*, p. 146.

p. 139   It's a point that Denise Riley makes beautifully: Denise Riley, *Time Lived, Without Its Flow* (London: Picador, 2019).

p. 139   'isolate you further …': Riley, *Time Lived, Without Its Flow*, p. 17.

p. 139   'No subject can easily be conceived as extinguished …': Riley, *Time Lived, Without Its Flow*, p. 62.

p. 140   'My best hope's to have a hallucination …': Riley, *Time Lived, Without Its Flow*, p. 52.

p. 140   'Self-pity': DH Lawrence, 'Self-pity', in *DH Lawrence, The Poems*, Vol. 1, edited by Christopher Pollnitz (Cambridge: Cambridge University Press, 2013), p. 405.

p. 141   'you have gone so far beyond me in suffering …': Philip Larkin, *The Selected Letters of Philip Larkin*, edited by Anthony Thwaite (London: Faber & Faber, 1992), p. 733.

p. 142   'If, as an adult, I ask myself whether I'd rather be alive than dead …': Galen Strawson, *Things That Bother Me: Death, Freedom, the Self, Etc.* (New York: The New York Review of Books, 2018), pp. 71–2.

p. 142   'happy, or in love, or looking forward to something' and 'My future life and experience …': Strawson, *Things That Bother Me*, p. 72.

p. 142   the smell of bread in the toaster: Thomas Nagel, *What Does It All Mean?* (Oxford: Oxford University Press, 1987), p. 93.

p. 145   'If we are to make sense of the view that to die is bad …': Thomas Nagel, *Mortal Questions* (Cambridge: Cambridge University Press, 2012), p. 4.

p. 147   Has the time come, to paraphrase Joan Didion, to let him go: Joan Didion, *The Year of Magical Thinking* (New York: Knopf, 2005).

p. 151   'of necessary failure': Jaco Barnard-Naudé, 'Hannah Arendt's Work of Mourning: The Politics of Loss, "The Rise of the Social" and The Ends of Apartheid', in *Remains of the Social: Desiring the Post-Apartheid*, edited by Maurits van Bever Donker, Ross Truscott, Gary Minkley and Premesh Lalul (New York: New York University Press, 2017), p. 129.

p. 151   a good example of what the sociologist Philippe Aries counterintuitively called a 'wild death': Philippe Ariès, *The Hour of Our Death* (New York: Knopf, 1981).

p. 153   a referring expression in disguise: Ben Dupré, *50 Ethics Ideas You Really Need to Know* (London: Hachette, 2013), p. 126.

p. 154   'we tend to build our practical identities around the existence of other people …': Michael Cholbi, *Grief: A Philosophical Guide* (Princeton, NJ: Princeton UN, 2021), p. 77.

p. 155   Living in the past, they argue, is not a 'feeble retreat' or an 'escape from reality': Chelsea Reid, Jeffrey Green, Stephen Short, Kelcie Willis, Jaclyn Moloney, Elizabeth Collison, Tim Wildschut, Constantine Sedikides and Sandra Gramling, 'The Past as a Resource for the Bereaved: Nostalgia Predicts Declines in Distress', *Cognition and Emotion*, vol. 35, no. 2 (2021), p. 263.

p. 155   'a coping mechanism for the bereaved': Jessica Blower and Rachael Sharman, 'To Grieve or Not to Grieve (Online)? Interactions with Deceased Facebook Friends', *Death Studies*, vol. 45, no. 3 (2021), p. 174.

p. 155   'nurtures social connectedness': Constantine Sedikides and Tim Wildschut, 'Nostalgia as Motivation', *Current Opinion in Psychology*, vol. 49 (2023), p. 2.

p. 155   'raises optimism': Constantine Sedikides and Tim Wildschut, 'Nostalgia: A Bittersweet Emotion That Confers Psychological Health Benefits', in *Wiley Handbook of Positive Clinical Psychology*, edited by Alex Wood and Judith Johnson (Hoboken, NJ: Wiley, 2016), p. 129.

p. 155   'to re-establish psychological homeostasis in the aftermath of distress': Reid et al., 'The Past as a Resource for the Bereaved', p. 259.

p. 155   'It is perhaps easier to die than ever tend to the dead?': Paul Stanbridge, *My Mind to Me a Kingdom Is* (Norwich: Galley Beggar Press, 2022), p. 217.

p. 156   'embodied sign-values': Phillip Vannini and Aaron McCright, 'To Die For: The Semiotic Seductive Power of the Tanned Body', *Symbolic Interaction*, vol. 27, no. 3 (2004), p. 309. 'Embodied sign-values' is a phrase that has stayed with me since I came across Vannini and McCright's article in 2022. The authors suggest that there are two competing frames or stories through which people interpret artificial tanning: a medical frame (whose proponents claim that extensive research has shown that prolonged exposure to UVA and UVB rays heightens the risk of skin cancer) and a seduction frame (a frame promoted by the tanning industry, popular magazines and 'beauty professionals', which equates tanning with physical attractiveness, and overall physical and mental well-being). For people who regularly tan their bodies, Vannini and McCright argue, the medical frame is less persuasive than the seductive frame, for 'the appearance of being healthy is more important' than any potential risk to physical health. The 'semiotic seductive power of the tanned body', the authors write, has significant 'value for its possessor' (328).

p. 157   but who exactly am I talking to: Nicci Gerrard, *What Dementia Teaches Us about Love* (London: Penguin, 2019), pp. 223–4.

p. 157   what Elisabeth Kübler-Ross calls the death-adjustment pattern: Elisabeth Kübler-Ross, *On Death and Dying* (New York: Macmillan, 1969).

p. 161 'Dear Bryan Wynter': W. S. Graham, 'Dear Bryan Wynter', in *New Collected Poems* (London: Faber, 2004), pp. 258–60.

p. 163 how they keep things together: Fiona Green, 'Achieve Further through Elegy', in *W. S. Graham: Speaking Towards You*, edited by Ralph Pite and Hester Jones (Liverpool: Liverpool University Press, 2004), p. 150.

p. 163 'What had been a more or less conventional romantic approach to nature …': Robert D. Richardson, *Three Roads Back: How Emerson, Thoreau, and William James Responded to the Greatest Losses of Their Lives* (New Jersey: Princeton University Press, 2023), p. 63.

p. 164 Is cancer, as the surgeon and writer Sherwin Nulan claims, 'amoral' and 'immoral'? Sherwin Nuland, *How We Die* (New York: Vintage, 1994), p. 210.

p. 164 'Ascribing a cunning deviousness to cancer …': Fergus Shanahan, *The Language of Illness* (Dublin: Liberties Press, 2020), p. 111.

p. 166 'The people leave and the things stay': John Fosse, *Morning and Evening* (Dallas, Texas: Dalkey Archive Press, 2015), p. 35.

p. 167 cracked every problem, starting, of course, 'with the problem of death': E. M. Cioran, *The Trouble with Being Born* (Harmondsworth: Penguin, 2012), p. 14.

p. 168 'We don't forget, but something *vacant* settles in us': Barthes, *Mourning Diary*, p. 227.

p. 169 Moments before he drank the hemlock that killed him … This account of Socrates learning to play a new melody on the flute is from E. M. Cioran's *Drawn and Quartered* (New York: Arcade Publishing, 2012), p. 82.

p. 170 'nothing can undo the fact that he lived …': Wilhelm Nero Pilate Barbellion, *The Diary of an Unfortunate Man* (Harmondsworth: Penguin, 2017), p. 301.

p. 170 'Darest thou now O soul, Walk out with me toward the unknown region …': Walt Whitman, *Leaves of Grass* (New York: Norton Critical Edition, 1973), p. 441.

In lieu of a conclusion: Four short postscripts

p. 173 'from lure to lure' and the air 'seemed golden with …': Francine Prose, 'Rubber Life', in *In The Stacks: Short Stories About Libraries and Librarians*, edited by Michael Cart (Woodstock, NY: The Overlook Press, 2002), p. 223.

p. 174 I learn that the local authority is planning further library cuts: Joe Locker, 'Nottingham May Have to "Accept Reality" of Library Closures', *The West Bridgford Wire* (13 August 2024).

p. 174 a flagship of civic renewal … a beacon that reaches a more varied audience: Ken Worpole, 'Why Libraries Matter for Britain', *The New Statesman* (20 July 2022).

p. 175 over 40 per cent of people believe it's pointless visiting friends and relatives with advanced dementia: BBC, 'Dementia Loved Ones "Benefit from Visits"', *BBC News* (1 January 2016).

p. 175 'Heartless as it may seem …': Claudia Mills, 'Duties to Ageing Parents', quoted in Bouke de Vries, '"I Am Your Son, Mother": Severe Dementia and Duties to Visit

Parents Who Can't Recognise You', *Medicine, Health Care and Philosophy*, vol. 23, no. 1 (2020), p. 18.

p. 175   pointless to continue such a relationship: Bouke de Vries, '"I Am Your Son"', p. 18.

p. 175   'proof we exist for other people': Annie Ernaux, *I Remain in Darkness* (London: Fitzcarraldo Editions, 1997), p. 51.

p. 175   The need for social contact, moreover, is greater for people living with dementia: Bouke de Vries, '"I Am Your Son"', p. 19.

p. 176   Dementia imposes barriers: Bouke de Vries, '"I Am Your Son"', p. 19.

p. 176   He might not recognize me 'in a narrowly cognitive sense': Janelle Taylor, 'On Recognition, Caring, and Dementia', *Medical Anthropology Quarterly*, vol. 24, no. 4 (2008), p. 329.

p. 176   'someone familiar perhaps': Taylor, 'On Recognition', p. 329.

p. 176   the simple act of upping and going …: Samuel Beckett, *More Pricks Than Kicks* (London: John Calder, 1993), p. 39.

p. 176   Like it does for the grieving characters in David Grossman's *Falling Out of Time*: David Grossman, *Falling Out of Time* (London: Jonathan Cape, 2014).

p. 177   perhaps even talking with them: Grossman, *Falling Out of Time*, p. 4.

p. 177   'a journey of memorialization': David James, *Discrepant Solace: Contemporary Literature and the Work of Consolation* (Oxford: Oxford University Press, 2019), p. 210.

p. 177   'If one had a pill that would "wipe out" the grief …': Michael Cholbi, *Grief: A Philosophical Guide* (Princeton, NJ: Princeton UN, 2021), p. 69.

p. 177   'route to our pasts …': Cholbi, *Grief*, p. 79.

p. 177   grief doesn't always progress in certain discrete stages … Arguably the most well-known death adjustment pattern is the five stages of grief (denial, anger, bargaining, depression and acceptance) as described by Elisabeth Kübler-Ross in *On Death and Dying* (New York: Macmillan, 1969).

p. 177   Reading, to paraphrase Fernando Pessoa, offered relief from life: Fernando Pessoa, *The Book of Disquiet* (London: Serpent's Tail, 2010), p. 5.

p. 177   helped transform my often vague and inexpressibly private anguish: Timothy Aubry, *Reading as Therapy: What Contemporary Fiction Does for Middle-Class Americans* (Iowa City: University of Iowa Press, 2011), p. 26.

p. 178   to have fallen out of time: David Grossman, *Falling Out of Time*, p. 62.

p. 178   'the time of the dead is, from now on …': Denise Riley, *Time Lived, Without Its Flow* (London: Picador, 2019), p. 83.

p. 178   for holding the living and the dead together: Max Porter, 'Introduction' to *Time Lived, Without Its Flow*, p. 9.

Reading and dementia: Poems for reading aloud

p. 179   'in measured familiarity': Catherine Robson, *Heart Beats: Everyday Life and the Memorized Poem* (New Jersey: Princeton University Press, 2015), p. 112.

INDEX

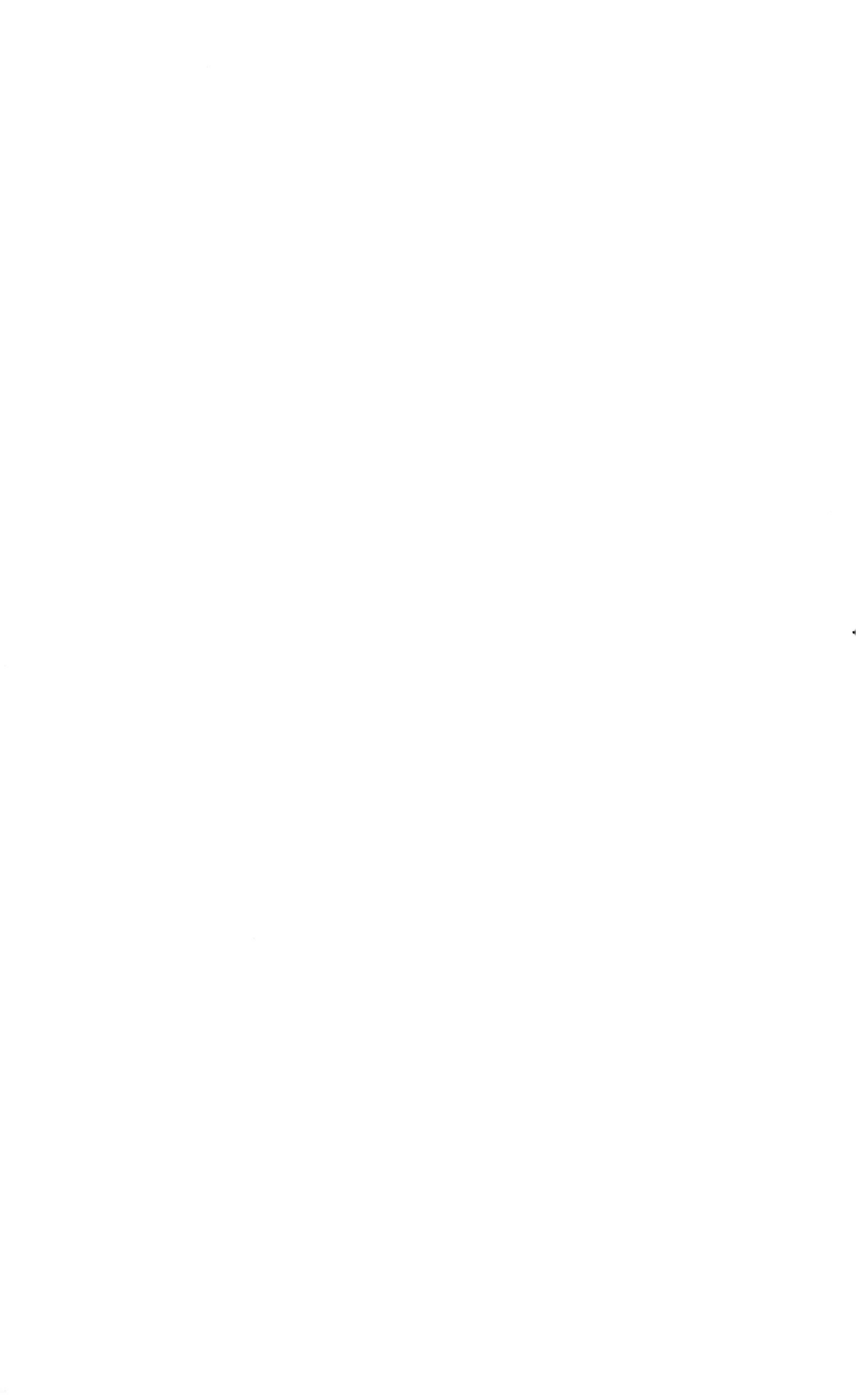